HEALTH Promotion
Spiritual HEALING

HEALTH Promotion Spiritual HEALING

Dr. Gwen Rose

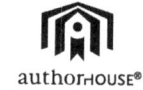
authorHOUSE®

AuthorHouse™
1663 Liberty Drive
Bloomington, IN 47403
www.authorhouse.com
Phone: 1-800-839-8640

LEWISHAM LIBRARY SERVICE	
Askews & Holts	20-Oct-2017
234.131	6

© 2012 by Dr. Gwen Rose. All rights reserved.

No part of this book may be reproduced, stored in a retrieval system, or transmitted by any means without the written permission of the author.

Published by AuthorHouse   2012

ISBN: 978-1-4678-9707-5 (sc)
ISBN: 978-1-4678-9708-2 (e)

Any people depicted in stock imagery provided by Thinkstock are models, and such images are being used for illustrative purposes only.
Certain stock imagery © Thinkstock.

This book is printed on acid-free paper.

Because of the dynamic nature of the Internet, any web addresses or links contained in this book may have changed since publication and may no longer be valid. The views expressed in this work are solely those of the author and do not necessarily reflect the views of the publisher, and the publisher hereby disclaims any responsibility for them.

Contents

Chapter One: Introduction and Context 1
    Introducing the Chapters and Sections 5

Chapter Two: The Holy Spirit, Power and Control—Who
    has the Power and Authority to Heal? 11
    Introduction 11
    The Church as an Organisation 12
    The Authority and Power of the Minister 13
        Charismatic Leaders 17
    Introducing the Holy Spirit as an Authority in Healing. 19
        The Holy Spirit as a Gift and Healing as a Gift 25
    Church Governance and Healing: The Minister as a
    Manager and Healer 26
        Selecting Spiritual Leaders in the Christian Churches 31
        Members with the Gift of Healing 35
        Becoming a Member and Learning to Heal 37
    Conclusion 38

Chapter Three: Suffering and Healing 39
    Introduction 39
    Suffering in Context 39
    Perceptions of Suffering 42
    Suffering and Faith 47
    The Difference between Illness and Disease as Suffering 52
    Drawing on Job as an Example of Suffering 57
    Suffering and the Casting out of Spirits 59
    Healing from the Suffering of Rejection 64
    Breaking the Generational Cycle of Suffering 68
    Conclusion 71

Chapter Four: Prayer as a Healing Activity 72
    Introduction 72
    Purpose of Prayer 73
    Prayer as Health Seeking Behaviour: How and When
    the Churches and Individuals Pray for Healing 76
    Prayer for Healing for Specific Illnesses 86
    Distance Healing versus Contact Healing 88
    Differences in How Prayer is Administered
    in the Churches 91
    Conclusion 95

Chapter Five: Laying on of Hands... 96
    Introduction 96
    Definitions and Use of the Terms within the Clinical
    and Popular Literatures 97
    The Practice of Laying on of hands or Therapeutic Touch 100
    Individual Experiences of Laying on of Hands 105
    Conclusion: Let them all come!...111

Chapter Six: Music for Worship and Healing 113
    Introduction 113
    Contextualising the Origins of Worship Music 114
    Mood Enhancing Medical Treatment: the Effects
    of Opioids...118
    Physiological Effects of Music 120
    Music as Therapy 123
    Conclusion 131

Chapter Seven: Conclusion 132
    Introduction 132
    The Vision..132
    The Process 133
    The Outcome: Similarities and Differences...........................135
    Conclusion and Reflections on the Study..............................139

References 145

About The Author

A Personal Journey

'God has brought me from a mighty long way'

Arriving at this point in my personal and professional life has been an interesting and laboured journey.
I was born of Jamaican parents in a small village district called Crawle River in Clarendon, Jamaica. As a young child when I compared my family to some of my peers at school, we were one of the less affluent families as we did not own a shop, a large plantation or large plot of land. There were large plots of 'family land' where we could graze the animals or use the produce, but as children we did not know who owned the land.

I regard myself as privileged because I was identified as 'bright' by my mother who sent me to private school when I was four years old. The law required children to attend state school when they were seven. My mother later informed me that she did not 'know what to do with me' so she sent me to school. I can remember going to school when I was very young and this was not state education as my parents had to pay. When my siblings and my peers were making a fuss about minor things such as fashionable clothes, I would stick my head in a book. My greatest pleasure was to complete the chores and read anything in print from the limited books that were available to the newspaper that was used to wrap items bought from the shop.

As I journeyed through my schooling and the education system in Jamaica, the only entertainment available to children was to go to church on Sunday and occasionally we would be chosen to participate in fundraising concert, held at one of the three churches in the village. We took it in turn to visit each church when there was a special occasion. Our family church was the Pentecostal (Church of God of Prophecy). The other two were the Baptist and the New Testament Church of God. Church life has been part of life for as long as I can remember.

My journey to Britain, like so many others, as analysed in Section 3, was to join my parents when I was a teenager in the early 1960s. My mother informed me many years later that she realized that she could not provide for all six of us to have education so she decided to take the opportunity to come to England in 1960.

I was devastated at having to leave high school. I passed the exams and had a scholarship to go high school and I missed the opportunity three times because my parents could not find money to buy books, uniform and meals. The scholarship covered the school fees only. As any young person who is displaced, I experienced a culture shock when I came to England. I had no friends, although friends who were not studious were not in my league. I was not allowed to go out to the cinema, nightclubs or any kind of entertainment except church. I did not mind too much because I could go to church and put a book on top of my bible and read the book instead of participating in all aspects of the service. My quest for knowledge was more intense than going out with friends. At the same time church life was ingrained in me. It became a part of me; it was a large part of my culture.

My personal faith became more real during the time that I was being sexually abused in my early teens by a male member of the church that I attended with my family. I was contemplating telling my parents although I thought he would deny this and my father would not believe me. I was convicted, converted and decided that I wanted to be baptized. It was as if God said 'I will rescue you from this wretched plight'. As soon as I announced that I wanted to be baptized the abuser stopped. At this point I believed that if I reported him my parents would believe me above him because I would not tell a lie now that I have become a born again Christian. I felt cleansed. Up to this point I felt guilty, unclean and generally like a sinner. Although I was a victim, as is usual with victims (the abused) in these situations, it felt that it was somehow my fault this was happening. Following my baptism I really felt and believe that God 'saved' me from the humiliation of being abused and probably being forced into a marriage that I did not want.

However, I soon realized that my own beliefs and understanding were very different from the majority of people in the church. One example of this is although I disagreed with the wearing of hats and other dress and activities rules, I complied to keep the peace. I was too busy being rebellious in my quest for knowledge.

Interestingly, after 30 years of protesting about the restricted mode of dress, my father said 'You will like the church now as they have changed the rules to allow women to wear makeup, jewels such as ear rings in the church.' By this time I had left the Church of God of Prophecy and there was no going back. My father was eternally disappointed as he would have liked one of his children to follow in his footstep in 'his' church. My first sister and I are both committed Christians, but we attended different churches.

My educational journey took me into the medical field, nursing, and later into teaching nurses, and health promotion. Following my Health Visiting training, I wanted to read with a purpose, so I registered for further study (not a degree). I did not think I was capable of studying for a degree. As my studies progressed I realized that I could become a teacher and study for a degree, so I combined the two. At 38 years I had finally achieved the goal to become a teacher which I set myself when I was four years old. Where do I go from here? I asked myself. The answer came loud and clear. 'Continue to pursue knowledge'. The next level of pursuing knowledge was a master's degree. I enrolled at a local University for a Master's Degree which incidentally was required for me to continue teaching. Four years after completing my Master's Degree I became bored and wanted to pursue more knowledge.

I stayed with my Christian beliefs although positive action in this area went on a back burner during the years when I raised my children and pursued my education.

Physical and emotional abuse from my mother and later at church has been contained by concentrating on the pursuit of knowledge. My mother

Dr. Gwen Rose

beat me and at times tied me to the pillar which was part of the foundation of our small one room house in Jamaica. My parents would probably call it discipline; I call it abuse, although I can understand this kind od violent discipline now as part of the legacy of slavery. This kind of discipline continued throughout my childhood. In my early teens I experienced sexual molestation from a senior male member of the church which I was unable to talk about because of the reaction I expected from my parents, and church family. I often heard adults talking about similar stories to my own (which I was not supposed to hear) about other children and it was always the fault of the children and not the adults. As I journeyed through my spiritual life, I realized that there were many emotional wounds that have not been healed. Healing was taught in the church, but this did not apply to me. I was too busy with earning a living, raising my family and pursuing an education to think about the scars from my childhood or from anyone else's for that matter.

The undeveloped potential of spiritual healing in health promotion became apparent to me during the years that I taught health promotion based on the Ewles and Simnett (1999) model of promoting health and healing, despite the fact that hospital chaplaincies appeared to provide a valuable service to patients in hospital. My curiosity was also fuelled by the apparent lack of knowledge of my fellow church members about their medical conditions and how to access health services on a personal level.

Their lack of desire for more medical knowledge was partly conditioned by their reliance on faith in God, which made too much concern with their bodily welfare almost into a questioning of God's providence. Compounding their failure to seek more information about their condition was their reluctance to give the doctor and the nurse information about the herbal (bush) remedies that they used. It was and continues to be common practice to use crushed garlic for high blood pressure and cerassie tea and ginger to help lower the blood sugar of diabetics. When I listened to the older people talk about their medical conditions it was like listening to a group of people that I knew nothing about. I realized that my knowledge of my own cultural heritage was extremely limited and I wanted desperately improve my own understanding as well as the understanding of my professional colleagues. Not only was my knowledge of my cultural heritage limited, but medical personnel, doctors, nurses, and physiotherapists also have limited knowledge of the cultural heritage of black and ethnic minority groups. Consequently the assessment and care that people from black and ethnic minority groups receive in the health and social care system is limited because of the lack of knowledge on both sides.

My journey into this research has also been prompted by the rejection that I have had from many people in terms of questioning my capability because of my cultural background. I was told by a senior lecturer (who was my mentor at the time) that I was writing West Indian English. This was the first time that anyone suggested this to me during some thirty years of studying, teaching and nursing in England. This really felt like an attack on my racial origin.

That discussion went further into a discussion of the political and social background which suggested that I was the victim (education product) of an era in Britain when teaching English in schools was not given a high profile. It was suggested that the mass import of labour from the Commonwealth countries, and the "political incorrectness" of old-fashioned grammar meant that teaching English in schools 'watered down' to make it easier for the masses. This coupled with my nurse training where writing about the patient and their care was more important than perfect English, meant that writing perfect English was not a priority. In consequence, by the time I trained as a teacher a large number of students had completed basic formal education including university education without the required 'standard' of written English. This was highlighted when these students arrived on a teacher's training course. Overseas students also found themselves in this category.

But, whilst feeling like a foreigner in White society, I also experienced rejection from the Black majority church and this illuminates the fact that I am truly between cultures. I am between cultures because of my education, which has informed my view of the church, and because of my age, caught between the older generation such as my parents and the younger generation such as my children. I have lived the shifting diasporic identity of Caribbean migrants to the UK described in section 3.

My sense of rejection was reinforced by the death of my mother in July 2002. I had realised that my mother was dying when I embarked on the journey of this research and the death of my mother made me more determined to complete this research as a tribute to myself, my mother and my family. The death of my mother made me realise that I was alone in my quest for knowledge and recognition in my own right. Not as a daughter, sister, mother, auntie teacher, friend, minister or any other role that I may assume in life. I wanted recognition for my work on my own terms.

In May 2006 my father died. I was surprised and pleased that he survived my mother by nearly four years. Following the death of my mother, I added to my isolation by refusing to continue the level of family responsibility that I had during my mother's lifetime and particularly during her illness. My siblings added to my isolation by their expectations of me to continue in the mothering role. They refused to communicate with me and I with them on a personal level. This isolation was compounded by the isolation I felt within the Black majority church I was studying. Although I learnt from previous research courses that researchers experience isolation during their research, I did not anticipate the extent of the isolation that I felt with the black majority Pentecostal church (COGIC). My expectations were that as a black researcher from a Pentecostal background, I would have an advantage that another person without similar background would not have.

After doing fieldwork for about 18 months, in some (most) situations I felt really isolated. I don't really belong anywhere as a person because I had to be very professional and mature in my approach to everything that I did. I had friends, but they were distanced, or rather I felt distanced from them. I made many changes in my personal and professional life prior to and at the beginning of this research and some changes were imposed on me. Throughout my life, I often felt very isolated and alone in my quest for new knowledge and information. Organizing time to concentrate on the thesis was a constant time-management juggling act and my time-management skills improved tremendously.

Why am I doing this at my age? I constantly asked myself.

On a day to day level the encouragement and inspiration were nonexistent. People have such busy lives and sometimes I had to make the same request five or six times before I got a response, and this could be very frustrating and I really wanted to give up. My supervisors were very supportive but I found it really hard to get local support. The fieldwork in the URC church went very well and the people were willing to volunteer to be interviewed and those who had been interviewed would ask me how the project was progressing. The fieldwork in the Pentecostal church did not go so well; however as the people were superficially friendly but not willing to volunteer to be interviewed.

I am still rather surprised at the reception that I received from the Pentecostal church. I started by approaching the Director of the Bible School on the premise that as the church houses an education department the majority of the church members have a commitment to education. The Bible School Director and the Pastor were very receptive on a superficial level, but I made several attempts to meet with both of them on a one to one basis with very little success. I overcame some of this isolation by joining a voluntary research group where all the group members were studying at PhD level and we had similar experiences. In contrast to my usually self sufficient approach to life, I had to learn to select appropriate people to ask and to keep asking for help. There are those who are willing to help but for reasons known best to themselves are not helping. The journey of this research means that I had to set new goals, make new friends and find new and different levels of support as an individual and a researcher.

This book is dedicated to my late parents Kenneth and Esmena Wallace, husband Leslie Rose, children Anthony and Katrina, grand children Joel and Xion and all those who supported me on this amazing journey.

Preface

This book addresses how 'Spiritual Healing' is administered in two Christian churches with similar doctrine but a different approach to how that doctrine is understood and practised. The divergence in eschatologies of the two different denominational congregations influences the way they integrate healing into their worship. There are also cultural differences in worship between them; the Black majority congregation engages in an animated charismatic style while the White majority practises in a more sedate and what may appear to an outsider to be a more passive style of worship. The study also examines the activities of prayer, laying on of hands and the use of music in the delivery of healing and as health promotion.

The study compares and contrasts the theology and practice of the two congregations and their understanding of spiritual healing. It is also shown that spiritual healing can be part of and complementary to the approach that medical and nursing professionals utilise in their practice. Recipients of spiritual healing whose health seeking behaviour straddles the medical and the spiritual approach may or may not use medicine as prescribed by health professionals. In the UK, people usually have access to both, unlike people in Developing countries who have limited access to modern medicine and have no choice but to make the best use of folk medicine, and faith healers in their health seeking behaviour practices. The study recommends that more mutual understanding may facilitate the support of faith groups for the work of the NHS recommended by recent government policy.

by Dr. Gwen Rose

Chapter One

Introduction and Context

The book explores the phenomena of spiritual healing in two Christian congregations who both practise it, and would acknowledge each other as recognizably Christian despite the differences in their understanding of what salvation means. The most important theological difference for the practice of healing are their eschatological beliefs about whether and how salvation means that Christians can claim all the biblical promises of healing now, or only at some point in an unknown future. This difference is further complicated by the cultural differences between the two congregations chosen for study. One is a Black majority congregation affiliated with the Church of God in Christ (COGIC), and engages in an animated, charismatic style of worship and healing which sometimes consciously patterns itself on the outpouring of the Holy Spirit at Pentecost. The other is a White majority congregation, affiliated with the United Reformed Church (URC) which engages in a more sedate style of worship and healing. The research addressed the growing engagement of health and social care professionals with faith and faith groups in health care in many communities and moreover the question of how spiritual healers and healing may be viewed as part of the health behaviour of individuals and communities as a whole.

To attempt this task involved researching a wide and confusing range of literatures; but this is perhaps not surprising. The great anthropologist Claude Lévi-Strauss (1966) talking about his research on healers in the South American forests suggests that the general method of healers in simple society is "*bricolage*".

Dr. Gwen Rose

A *bricoleur* is the French word for the kind of village odd-job or handyman who keeps every odd nut, screw or piece of wood or metal he can lay his hands on, and if anything breaks down in the village he can generally fix it from the old spare parts that he has hoarded.

Lévi-Strauss said that the general method of primitive healers in simple societies was like that of those *bricoleurs*: basically, use anything that works. A few herbs, animal grease, magic mushrooms, prayers, music, manipulation; and if it ever seems to work on anything once, remember to try it again just in case. Above all, put on a serious, confident air to make the clients believe you know what you are doing, since their belief is half the battle—the placebo effect IS very powerful—taking a placebo does produce a better outcome than doing nothing.

Lévi-Strauss contrasted this primitive method with modern science, (which he believed was guided by Cartesian rationality). The modern sociology of science, however, from the detailed historical examination by Thomas Kuhn (1970) of how slowly and partially Einstein's theory of relativity spread in the 1920s, to Michael Mulkay's (1991) painstaking laboratory ethnographies, shows us that actually scientists are still doing *bricolage*, except they call it by the politer philosophical term "pragmatism".
Lévi-Strauss (1963) in his essay 'The effectiveness of Symbols' himself maps the practices of the Cuna *nele* (healer) onto contemporary psychoanalytic practice, while Littlewood and Dein (2000), follow others in examining whether this is a kind of general comparison between "shamanism" and medical science, or whether it is just saying that psycho-analysis is not better than faith-healing. My research shows that in the world of spiritual healing, *bricolage* and the use of symbols through faith is still practised. When we feel sick, we want whatever might work. Indeed this thesis is itself an example of *bricolage*, collecting material from everywhere and showing how it works together in the world of ideas.

The research examines to what extent spiritual healing is complementary to medical practice and what are the limitations and successes of spiritual healing. In the NHS Plan, (Department of Health 2000:106), the Government directive for the health service of the millennium embraces partnership. Health Service Trusts and Local Authorities have moved towards working in partnership with minority ethnic and faith groups to deliver the new NHS and social care plan, although more recently Wright (2007) has warned about the burdens that might be placed on nurses by a reduction in the number of hospital chaplains. It will be suggested that, although it is not necessary for NHS staff fully to understand all aspects of spiritual care, it is necessary for those who deliver health and spiritual care to have a proper understanding of it and be more prepared to work in a collaborative approach with each other at different levels of delivery.

The study a) Explored the perception of spiritual healing in church goers in the two congregations; b) Observed healing services in a White majority and a Black majority Christian church; c) Explored healing in the context of culture of the church and the ethnic origin of the church goers.

These objectives do not include assessing empirically the efficacy of any form of spiritual healing. There exists a limited clinical literature which has attempted this (c.f. Breslin et al, 2008) which is presented briefly in section one. There is no definitive evidence of the effects of spiritual healing such as might be provided by a double-blind controlled experiment, but examining it helps to show how it would be impossible to conduct a controlled survey, even if it were ethical to do so. Indeed it is impossible to conceive how someone might pray for the healing of only a selection of people without all the prayers thereby, being rendered insincere—and how would an observer measure sincerity? The present study, therefore, does not affect the overall tendency of the existing research literature to suggest the indications of any overall or general effectiveness of prayers for health are inconclusive, and it reinforces the notion that further research is best concentrated on reaching a better understanding of the different aspects of prayer and healing in coping with adverse stress in specific illness contexts.

This study starts from the discourse on the promotion of health in contemporary British society and in particular, the more inclusive approach of recent years which has involved previously relatively excluded groups like the disabled, Black and other minority ethnic people in the planning and delivery of health and social care services. Since 1997 under the Labour Government, this inclusive approach has led to a new open-ness to faith based initiatives. The spiritual domain, however, has been given little importance among the five approaches presented in the dominant Ewles and Simnett (1999) model for the promotion of health. This model was used by the present writer and other colleagues to deliver health promotion courses to nurses and other health and social care professionals over several years, but seemed increasingly to place little importance on the role of spirituality in health promotion. Her own African-Caribbean culture cultural heritage also appeared as an important omission.

To remedy these gaps in the discourse of health promotion, looking at a white majority culture as well as Afro-Caribbean culture, it was decided to use an ethnographic approach. Two specific congregations were chosen for the investigation, one belonging to the Church of God in Christ (COGIC) and one to the United Reform Church (URC). The research method set out to interrogate the perceptions of church attendees, through semi-structured interviews, and through participant and non-participant observation. Since I was bringing much of my own experience to the work, I realised it was necessary to be rigorous in applying autobiographical method as emphasised most recently by Muncey (2010). I have therefore used my life experiences as evidence, and in discerning and shaping the formulation of the hypotheses.

This is an illustration of the author's personal journey to the beginning of research, contextualising what follows. The journeys through the data collection and the writing of the thesis have also had a profound effect on my view of the world, both spiritual and academic. I am not, however, using my own experience as my primary data as Muncey's (2010) autobiographical approach to auto-ethnography suggests, as it was important for me to try step outside my own world in order to create a distance from the data during the collection process as well as during the writing up phase.

Although I share the common bond of socio-cultural and spiritual identity with the research topic and the respondents, the methodology chosen is not dependent on autobiography. I also share the ambivalence towards biographical enterprise as scientific method in itself as expressed by McAdams and West (1997). The methodological principles of auto-ethnography guide, it is to be hoped, my critical reflection throughout the process (c.f. Spry 2001). The methodological approach of observation, interview and reflexivity is one with which I am familiar since as I have used it throughout my professional life. It seemed appropriate to build on a familiar methodology in the same way that my personal, professional and academic skills have been developed throughout the process of producing this thesis.

The following hypotheses guided the questions for the interviews:
a) Spiritual healing may be perceived by church-attending actors in illness and health behaviour as a strong factor in the success of delivering health
b) People's compliance with formal and informal health programmes are closely related to their belief systems.
The discussion of themes elicited from the data is given in chapters 1-5 and the chapters are summarized in the final chapter as a conclusion.

Introducing the Chapters and Sections

The original thesis comprises 10 chapters. Presented here is a summary of chapters 2-4 as section one—three and chapters one, and six to ten is presented as chapters one—seven. In section one the literature review is presented in sections; firstly, on health and health promotion models, next on illness behaviour and health seeking behaviour, thirdly, an exploration of the complexity of conceptions of spirituality and spiritual healing within a context of culture, the spiritual concepts of health, and folk medicine. Finally, the discourse of sociology of religion provides a framework to look at the development and history of the Pentecostal movement in Britain and to contrast it with the URC.

Section two describes the methodology, how the research used an ethnographic approach based on Brewer (2000), which includes participant and non—participant observation, and semi-structured interviews to collect qualitative data with the aim of using triangulation in the analysis of the data. Two churches were chosen as research sites and their Ministers were approached with the proposal and asked for permission to conduct fieldwork. After starting the observations the researcher then requested that she should personally address the church attendees at the Pentecostal church as there had been no expression of interest in the study topic that was made directly to the researcher.

Following the announcement at the URC church meeting, the researcher received several offers of interest in the study topic. The church meeting was an open meeting that could be attended by anyone who attended the church, although only church members were allowed to vote on topics that required a vote. The Pentecostal church has a more closed committee of all church members.

The interviews were audio taped and then transcribed. The respondents had the option to withdraw from the study at any time during the volunteering, interview and post interview phase. They signed a consent form and were asked to read the transcript, ask for a copy of the audiotape and make comments on the contents of the transcript when they signed the consent form, and again when the transcribing process was completed. None of the respondents took the opportunity to request the audiotapes or to read the transcript.

On examining models of data analysis such as discourse analysis (Brewer 2000, Miles and Huberman 1994) and McCracken's (1988) model, the latter was chosen after my learning to use the NVivo coding framework and linking this with the different stages of analysis that were required for this ethnographic study.

McCracken's model describes five stages of analysis and these stages can be carried out using the NVivo software package (Bazeley and Richards 2000). The stages are

1. Coding utterances in the data. NVivo allocates the name of attributes or nodes where a term is selected and NVivo identifies the number of times this word or group of words appear in the data (interviews, observations, notes)
2. This stage develops the attributes according to the evidence in the data or the context in which they are used in the data.
3. This stage examines the interconnection between the attributes and the literature
4. This stage subjects the observations generated from the previous stages to further scrutiny.
5. The final stage selects patterns and themes as they appear in several interviews and subjects them to another level of analysis. (c.f. Brewer 2000: 42,)

Section 3 describes the people, the congregations, their practices and their background and present circumstances drawing on both fieldwork and written sources. The observations and interviews revealed aspects of the Pentecostal church providing knowledge of such matters as their order of service, the Lord's supper (communion), the fasting service on the first Sunday of each month, and weekday gatherings where the elderly (especially women) meet for prayer and fellowship. For many retired people their contribution to the community is through their prayer group. These groups are open to everyone who wishes to attend but there is usually a core group of older people who attend regularly. The chapter also explores the historical context of the churches, their doctrine, the hierarchy and physical aspects of the healing environment.

Chapter two describes the power and control of the minister, the organizational cultures of the churches as religious and charitable bodies and compares them with the organizational culture of secular organizations. It argues that the authority structure is related to the theology of the Holy Spirit, and this governs religious practices such as 'speaking in tongues' as well as spiritual healing, The discussion outline the relationship of theology to issues of power, authority and control in the church as an organization (c.f. Keay 1987). Although there are overarching commonalties, to provide an in-depth view of the differences, aspects of each congregation will be examined separately. The church as an organization has similarities with other caring organizations where 'care is fundamental to the pact involving human beings and where care is more than a service industry.' (Henderson and Atkinson 2003:7). Within both churches there are many sub-cultural traditions but the main contrast examined here is between the overall black majority and white majority from a cultural and racial perspective. In addition to this, the organizational and political culture is also examined.

Chapter three describes evidence from the data about suffering as overt or covert pain. This pain can be the result of physical, psychological, emotional or spiritual pain. The data shows persons who are suffering with physical, emotional or mental imbalances which could be short term or long term suffering. In any one human experience, there may be a mixture of more than one element of suffering. One person can share another person's suffering by empathizing with them, because they have experienced a similar situation or actually sharing the situation with them.

The suffering of one family member radiates to other family members in varying degrees.

Drawing on the literature on suffering, the concept of suffering in the bible and the respondents' perception of suffering, it will be shown the form of suffering follows the cultural perception of the person who is suffering and others who see them as suffering. The history of the churches, the experience of folk medicine, and the degree of spiritual and psychological support interact to shape the subjective experience of suffering.
Perception of demonic possession is included in this chapter from the healing perspective whereas it is included in chapter 4 from the cultural and belief system perspective. It is important to note that concern with the concept of pain and suffering runs throughout the thesis.

Chapter four explores prayer as one of the main health seeking behaviours and health promotion activities used in distant healing and contact healing in the two churches in the study. In the Pentecostal congregation prayer for healing is not separated from prayer for repentance, sanctification, justification and becoming a born again Christian. In the URC prayer for healing is focused during intercessory prayers during normal Sunday services and there is also a healing service where the whole service if focused on healing and concludes with prayer and the 'laying of hands' by the minister and elders for anyone who wishes to take this opportunity to have a focused prayer. The literature, observation and other research literature show that research into the effects of prayer is inconclusive. They neither proves or disproves that prayer is effective as a tool in spiritual healing. It can therefore be concluded that more research is needed for a better understanding of the different aspects of prayer and healing in coping with adverse stress and illness.

Chapter five examines the 'laying on of hands' as an approach to using touch as technique in spiritual healing and also explores the concept of laying of hands as the biblical practice of the healing touch used in the medical/nursing field and the healing touch used in complementary therapies. There is also an exploration as to why and how using touch and the energy field of the spiritual healer can be regarded as an environment for healing and the possibility of transferring illness to the healer from the person seeking healing or transferring from the person seeking healing to the healer. Both churches practise the laying of hands for healing as directed in the bible where the elders are called upon to lay hands on the sick, in a manner similar to the "therapeutic touch" discussed by Hallett (2004).

Chapter six discusses the music observed in the services observed in both churches where music for worship is prominent as background music as well as music where some or all the congregation takes part. It explores the differences in the music and the effect of the different kind of music that is played in each church. It will also examine the provision of music as one of the departments within the Pentecostal church. It will also analyse the views expressed by respondents about music and its therapeutic potential using the theory of Harvey (2005) which suggests there are four distinct ways in which the brain responds to music. They are cognitive, affective, personal and transpersonal. In other words we respond to music by feeling the music with our emotions (cognitive, affective), by noticing the effect on our heart rate and breathing (physical) and feeling the connection of God (transpersonal) though music. It is noted earlier in the thesis that empirical analyses of responses to music provide a methodological model for understanding connections between physiological and psychological responses.

Chapter seven provides a brief discussion, conclusion and recommendations. The finding of the research has highlighted that there is a gap between the church and the NHS in delivering a collaborative and a partnership service to patients as directed by Government white papers such as Saving Lives, Our Healthier Nation (Department of Health 1999), The NHS Plan (Department of Health 2000) and Legislations such as The NHS and Community Care Act (Department of Health 1992). A strategy which takes account of the substance of religious faith and practice rather than just seeing it as one extra counselling resource is needed.

The findings give a clear indication that church attendees in both organizations uses the opportunity to seek healing and use this as complementary to medical and nursing care. Indicated recommendations are made that more research is needed, and that the churches, especially the Black Pentecostals, should familiarize themselves with the discourses

Dr. Gwen Rose

and practices of academic research, so that they can present their own contributions fairly and cogently, and understand and engage with critiques made by those of other or no faith traditions. Increased interaction between congregations from different ethnic traditions can only improve such understanding.

Chapter Two

The Holy Spirit, Power and Control—Who has the Power and Authority to Heal?

Introduction

This chapter describes the power and control of the minister, the organizational cultures of the churches as religious and charitable bodies and compares these with the organizational culture of secular organizations. It argues that the authority structure is related to a theology of the Holy Spirit, and this governs religious practices (such as 'speaking in tongues' as well as spiritual healing), following the discussion of the relation of theology to issues of power, authority and control in the church as an organization. Although there are overarching commonalties, aspects of each congregation will be examined separately to provide an in-depth view of the differences. The church as an organization has similarities with other caring organizations where "care is fundamental to the pact involving human beings" and where it seems as more than a service industry (Aldgate and Dimmock 2003). Within both churches there are many sub-cultural traditions but the main contrast examined here is between the black majority and white majority cultural and racial perspectives. In addition to this, the organizational and political culture of healing is also examined.

The terms 'pastor' and 'minister' are used interchangeably: COGIC and other Pentecostal churches use the term pastor to identify the director or chief executive of the local church while URC uses the term minister for the same purpose. The word 'leader' describes those in a leadership position, be it only for the purpose of one meeting or a subsection of the organization. This role can only be sanctioned by a minister with overall managerial responsibility for the church at local, national or international level.

The professional role of the minister in the process of administering spiritual healing is explored in two parts regarding power and authority: (a) the power and authority of the minister versus the power and authority of the Holy Spirit and (b) the power and authority of the minister as part of the wider church as an organization, which is compared with organizational theory in the world of business. The historical development of the churches was detailed in chapter 4. This chapter continues with an analysis of the authority afforded to the Holy Spirit by the church and the extent to which the pastor/minister exercises his own human authority and to what extent the authority of the Holy Spirit.

The word 'pastor' has been selected from the data as it is indicative of the local leader who makes ultimate decisions as to how the organization function on a spiritual and secular level. He does this as an individual or in consultation with other appointed leaders who serve the local churches and the wider national and international aspect of the organizations. Ephesians 4 identifies the titles of the leaders who were selected to lead the early church and give instructions as to how people should function in the roles of apostles, prophets, evangelists and teachers. This list does not include elders although in Acts, Chapter 20, v 17, Paul sent to Ephesus to call the elders of the church and James instructs the suffering and the sick to call for the elders of the church to 'pray over him and anoint him with oil. Paul also identifies the gifts, including healing that are attached to these roles. The roles and gifts are often interchangeable.

The Church as an Organisation

The two churches in the study as organizations rely on the power of the Holy Spirit to lead all its activities. Meetings are separated into two kinds: those for dealing with the business of the church and those for worship and healing. At church 'business' meetings, organizational and financial issues are discussed while during worship meetings worship and healing are foremost and organizational and financial issues of secondary importance. All church meetings in these congregations begin with prayer and are led by the minister or acting minister. Church meetings, then, are the only business meetings that always open and close with prayer. Other organizational meetings do not necessarily begin or close with prayer.

All organizations and institutions have the power and control system of a hierarchy, a bureaucratic system and an organization culture as outlined in tables 2 and 3 in chapter 4. Christian churches have the added caveat of the power, control and leading of the Holy Spirit. Power and control are based on biblical interpretation by the head (leader) of the organization to suit the leader or the group and those from within the group who reject opposition from outside the group. This suggests that power and control of healing cannot be based on basic human ability alone. There is a belief that there are some supernatural forces in action for spiritual healing to take place. There are also myriad cultural traditions within both churches but the main contrast to be examined here is between the black majority and white majority cultural and racial perspectives and the organizational and political culture within these churches. Many religious organisations share the belief that there is a divine presence which surpasses all human understanding and allow themselves to be guided by their spiritual leaders. The Christian traditions in this study regard the Holy Spirit as the divine agent that mediates the Father and the Son.

The Authority and Power of the Minister

In both churches observed in this study, the minister, as a leader, has authority when it is legitimised by the denomination and the local congregation. Ideas of legitimate authority also depend on the interpretation of scripture and the doctrine of the Holy Spirit (c.f. Muser 1992). All URC ministers have to demonstrate their leadership abilities on paper as well as in practice. The same is true for younger COGIC ministers who have been appointed in the past ten to twenty years as the older ministers, who were appointed in the early days following their migration to Britain, retire or become too old to function as leaders. COGIC has fewer full time ministers than URC. This may have some relationship to the availability of training that is acceptable to the church authorities and the few ministers' training colleges that are specific or suitable for Pentecostal ministers. The number of ministers in the URC—like the membership—has decreased considerably in recent years where it more commonplace for one minister to have responsibility for more than one church (United Reformed Churches, 2008). Yet the number of members has increased in the Pentecostal churches like COGIC (Thomas-Juggan, 2000).

Using NVIVO software on collected data to select and code, I have charted the occurrences of the word 'pastor' and 'minister' in the interviews and observational material as I have described in chapter 3. This was prompted by the comment of the minister in the extract below, who was unable to gain access to a hospital ward to visit a patient because he failed to introduce himself as a relative or a trained minister. This instance highlights the minister's power and authority within the church and the wider society.

The word 'pastor' is mentioned 108 times in eleven documents and the word 'minister' is mentioned 132 times in seventeen documents. COGIC and other black majority churches refer to their leader as Pastor and URC as Minister. The terms have similar connotations in the church and in the wider society. In the words of one minister *"I decided to become a minister formally because I was refused entry to a hospital ward to see someone I was working closely and praying with. I was told that only approved ministers are allowed to visit"*.

The above extract indicates that the approved minister is accepted by virtue of his status or power and authority in the church and by virtue of his status in the community and the wider society. The minister is accepted as part of the healthcare team as there is an understanding that qualified church ministers have a certain level of professionalism, trust, knowledge and the competence to respect other professionals who are caring for the patient. It is also accepted that the minister can bring some level of comfort and by extension, healing to the patient.

For the purpose of this chapter the terms pastor and minister are interchangeable in that they both refer to the locally-situated person responsible for the decision making processes in the local church. He (or she) is the person to whom the congregation looks for guidance on spiritual matters as well as for church governance. This individual also has a prominent position in the community and in places where the sick reside such as hospitals and care homes. The above extract makes clear that other than relatives, healing or pastoral institutions such as hospitals and hospices will only recognize approved ministers of religion as part of the 'professional healing team'. The wider societies also accept ministers of religion as professionals since they have undertaken a course of study or apprenticeship to become approved (professional) ministers.

The terms 'pastor', used by COGIC, and 'minister', used by URC, have biblical origins and describe those who have been selected as leader and who possesses special qualities. To be called pastor or minister, the individual is required to undertake a period of training or apprenticeship commitment, and discipleship within their organization/denomination to prepare them for the role. They will also have expressed a vocational calling and also possess the approval and acceptance of the wider and local church.

The main contrast that I will examine here is that existing between the differing perspectives of the black majority and white majority churches. There is evidence that the two churches differ in the disputes and fission explored by Calley (1965) who conducted groundbreaking research on the Pentecostal movement in England. However, Calley terms the Pentecostal movement a 'sect', a term limited in its usefulness given its negative connotations and its implication that the 'Pentecostalists' are distinctly set apart from the mainstream churches. Calley's linguistic choice when describing Black majority churches defines those with different cultural practices as 'aliens' despite their presence in British society. My research brings me to the opinion that Calley's interpretation of the worship methods and organizational structure of Black majority Pentecostal churches is personal rather than rigorously researched. He fails to give an overview of the various cultural traditions that exist in British Black majority Christian churches. Hill (1973) describes the structure of the black churches as resting on 'charismatic legitimacy'. It is a fact that charismatic leadership and an animated style of worship is a common denominator among black majority churches. Hill (1973) unpacks the term 'charismatic legitimacy' by outlining its constituent elements which include persuasive force, compliance, obedience and cultural patterns of how authority is acknowledged and respected. For example, older persons in the black majority church earn respect by reason of their age. This is also a cultural norm amongst black people. Status also entitles individuals to a certain level of respect which has nothing to do with age. Therefore, a pastor, elder, evangelist, and Sunday school teacher are revered as God's chosen ministers. If the individual holds a position in the church *and* also has seniority in age then they are doubly respected. Any dispute with God's minister must be legitimized by the Holy Spirit and a more senior minister.

Power, status and authority in one setting do not give the person equal status in another. African and West Indian immigrants may leave behind high rank in their own country taking up lower positions in Britain, thus experiencing loss of status as displaced people. As some of the critics of liberation theology discussed by McGovern (1989) suggest, a move to another country may be a move towards a new form of servitude and less authentic freedom. Many sought to replace their loss of status and new form of servitude with positions (office) in the church or deny the importance of achieving high status.

Within the Black community in Britain there is often an assumption that society runs on an assumption of white superiority and black inferiority. This stems in part from the fact that although black people have been present in Britain since Roman times they were only officially recognized by the 1991 British census (Raleigh and Balarajan 1994). Therefore as a people their visible presence in Britain is thought by most to be relatively new. Historically they are not new to the country but their visible presence is relatively new (c.f. Hiro 1991, Ahmad, 1993). Black people's relatively new presence in Britain as well as their relatively small numbers means that they possess less political power than the white majority. In recent years with Britain entering the European Community, black people have yet again been placed in the underclass as they struggle to compete against people from the European mainland to obtain work and to be recognized as a valuable part of the work force and not just fit for menial tasks. With little recognized status in the world of work it is not surprising that members of this marginalized community seek refuge in the (Pentecostal) church, an organization where Black people are often in positions of power and control (Toulis, 1997).

Charismatic Leaders

Charismatic leaders are associated with charismatic gifts within Pentecostalism as described by Anderson (2004) in the tradition broadly derived from Weber's (1947) discussion of the role of charisma in legitimation. As with all self-legitimating phenomena whose explanations are contested, charismatic leaders and gifts are sometimes seen in negative light and can indeed be viewed as signs of the demonic in the official church. Warrington (2008) asserts that Pentecostals believe that charismata gifts are not given on merit but are the result of the Grace of God.

The word 'charismatic' has also been used in the context of organisations outside the denominational or classical Pentecostals. Charismatic leadership, in the Pentecostal tradition, however, relates to leaders with special potential and authority guided by grace and the authority of the 'higher self'. However, no leader has power or authority unless the group that they lead legitimizes their authority with a nomenclature that is accepted by the group. In Biblical terms pastors, teachers, apostles, bishops are names used to denote people of high authority and with leadership qualities. The Charismatic movement has brought focus on the doctrine of the Holy Spirit and how to express this in their worship (McGrath 1995). Although each congregation (URC and COGIC) understand and practise the operation of the Holy Spirit in different ways, they both view it as the final authority that guides their leaders.

A lively style of worship that involves singing, shouting, dancing, crying and laughter in the belief that this is under the authority of the Holy Spirit is the norm in Pentecostal churches like COGIC. It would be difficult for URC ministers who did not have similar beliefs to lead a church with a Pentecostal style of worship. Although URC accept the visitation of the Holy Spirit, speaking in tongues and give emphasis to Pentecost, their worship style under the guidance of the Holy Spirit is usually more sedate, although there are some URC congregations which adopt a charismatic style of worship.

Richardson and Bowden (1999) explain charismatic phenomena as the grace dimension of the Christian church as distinguished from the institutional and hierarchical dimensions. This indicates a holistic approach to the church; where a grace orientated church is part of the hierarchical and the institutional church. The Pauline letters appears to confirm this concept in Corinthians, Romans and Ephesians. For many believers there is more overt evidence of charismatic leadership in the black majority churches and more evidence of institutional hierarchy in the URC and white majority churches. Although the Pentecostal churches are more spontaneous in their style of worship, this does not mean that they are more grace orientated in their belief and leadership style than the URC. Charismatic and divine leadership is sometimes confused with animation and spontaneity according to Beckford (2000: 174-7).

Hill (1973) argues that no leader can be labelled charismatic unless he is credited with the possession of such powers by his followers, yet charisma is not necessarily concerned with leadership although it is about authority. The power and authority of the minister is occasionally challenged, especially when there is a conflict of opinion about church doctrine and moral principles which are interpreted and applied by a particular group. The power of the Holy Spirit is also often challenged because it is only operational when applied to actions of a person who is deemed to be 'filled with the Holy Spirit'. There is a relationship between the theology of the Holy Spirit, and the religious practices and manifestations such as 'speaking in tongues' as well as spiritual healing. Embodying this theology are the issues of power, authority and control in the church as an organization.

Although there are biblical examples of women using them as well as men using spiritual gifts, few women occupy the position of minister who manages the organization locally and nationally (c.f Foster and Foster 1987). This is despite church membership in both Pentecostal and URC congregations, as in the majority of churches, being predominantly female. In the researched church (URC) the eldership consists of four females and one male and is led by a male minister.

The local URC church meeting is held every two months and is always chaired by the male minister. The elders (majority female) meet fortnightly for prayer and to discuss church governance and membership issues. They also have some pastoral function as well as participating in serving communion and healing. By contrast in COGIC, women are not allowed to serve communion, although they may take a lead role in many other activities such as worship and healing services, prayer, and the youth and Sunday school departments. The URC are divided about the role of women ministers: while some local churches allow women to serve communion others do not. The matter is usually decided according to the church's tradition. For instance, if the church has been led by a minister and his wife acting as equal partners then in the event of one partner's death, the other will assume full ministerial responsibilities (including serving communion) with the full support of the local church members and sanctioned by the Church Council or Synod.

Introducing the Holy Spirit as an Authority in Healing.

According to Christian tradition, the Holy Spirit is a distinct person within Triune God, the Father, Son (Jesus) and Holy Spirit. It is used to designate the third person of the divine Trinity (Gaunton 1997). Christian doctrine understands the Holy Spirit as a divine agent. (Richardson and Bowden 1999:262). In Christian tradition, healing is dependent on the Holy Spirit and biblical passages are often used to support this. Not all Christian Theology shares in relating doctrines of the Holy Spirit to a physical healing and charismatic experience; although Moltman (1997) postulates that the experience of the Spirit means a renewal of the soul and sometimes of the body. The Christian hope and claim for healing is directed towards a new creation of all things through the resurrection of Jesus Christ. The authority of the Holy Spirit to heal is a combination of the renewal processes at all stages of life and is also derived from historical sources. One of the key words relating to Pentecostals is Power—'The Power of the Holy Spirit' Warrington (2008) advocates that the Power of the Spirit empower, transforms and guides believers and that the giving and receiving of this Power is evidenced in the many manifestations of the Holy Spirit before and after the outpouring at Pentecost and later at Azusa Street.

Evidence of the Holy Spirit in operation is reported in the testimonies of eye-witnesses at Azusa Street (Anderson (2004). The renewed outpouring of the Spirit (the first outpouring that was regarded as newsworthy) took place in the West in North America at the Red River Church in 1899 and then again in Kentucky two years later, swiftly followed by the Azusa Street outpouring in 1906. After Azusa Street further Pentecostal groups developed not just in Europe, but also in Hong Kong in 1907 and Shanghai in 1910 and others grew up in the East and West. As noted in chapter 4 of the complete thesis, Black Pentecostalism arrived in Britain during the 1950s to 1970s. This was the same time as charismatic movements began to grow in mainline denominations in USA, Europe and other parts of the world (Steel 2005). Although the Holy Spirit was manifested in practical terms by the outpouring at Pentecost, some theologians see the healing brought about by the Spirit to be framed in terms of freedom and salvation from bondage. The manifestation of the Holy Spirit is illustrated on many occasions in the Old and the New Testaments which includes the appointment of elders by Moses to assist his leadership and to enable Elijah and Elisha to function charismatically (Warrington 2008)

Christian doctrine understands the Holy Spirit as a divine agent, which brings trans-creation of the human cosmic liberation (Richardson and Bowden 1999:262). 'The Spirit of God is the basic source of life' (Gaunton 1997). Beckford (2000) and Warrington (2008), all define the 'power of the Spirit as the ability to reckon with superhuman forces, the Spirit of God being the supreme spiritual force in the Universe'. Gaunton (1997) discusses many instances of the operation of the Holy Spirit in these tasks and responsibilities in the Old and New Testament. Muddiman (2001) asserts that in the letter to the Ephesians, Paul makes reference to the Spirit world, beyond the world of ordinary sense perceptions which should be the focus of the people as a church. The ecclesiology of the Pentecostal church is often related directly to the Spirit. In Eastern orthodoxy, Zizioulas (1985) writes about the presence of the Holy Spirit as an authority in the church in whatever expression it appears in different cultures and times. The church was instituted by Christ but constituted by the Holy Spirit. In the Pentecostal churches the appearance of charismatic gifts, rather than the sacraments is evidence that the spirit is present. Both Eastern Orthodox and Pentecostals are less Christocentric in their language about the Church, preferring to speak of the presence of the Spirit as bringing about power and authority in the church. Those who lead healing services or worship usually base their beliefs on the discerning spirit of Jesus and His power to heal and are not too worried that the question of how it works is mysterious. Hollenweger (1972) reports one American Pentecostal describing her experience of the baptism of the Holy Spirit and healing as the high times in her life. She said 'I really lived in another world for a solid week. It seems as if I hardly touch the ground. I was so lost in God and heavenly things. As Village (2005) points out, this does not mean they reject empirical research on the process and outcomes of spiritual healing activities, but they do not depend on this for the validation (which anyway it does not really offer).

Although the Spirit transforms believers according to Warrington (2008), when there is a dispute, healing can take place when the Holy Spirit is allowed to operate in a given situation. The Pentecostal churches teach and claim to practice spiritual healing, yet, it is not practised in a way that can be easily understood in the case of a dispute. All disputes cause some psychological pain, rejection is often experienced and the individual who is being challenged may feel their position or opinion is undermined. These hurtful feelings can fester and become deep wounds. Calley (1965) explains that in Pentecostal churches such as Church of God in Christ (COGIC) breaches are difficult to heal because when there is dispute between a church leader and a person who challenges the leader the correct response is to withdraw from 'a church whose doctrine is regarded as false'. This course of action is apparently sanctioned by 2 Thessalonians 3: 'Now we command you brethren, in the name of our Lord Jesus Christ, that ye withdraw yourself from every brother who walk disorderly, and not of the tradition he received us.' If a peace maker or arbitrator is appointed to help resolve dispute, he has to take sides or appeal to the disputants to bury their differences. The peacemaker is described in the Sermon on the Mount in Matthew as blessed. Calley (1965) implies that the peacemaker cannot afford to be seen to causing further dissension. He therefore has a ritualistic role to play rather than a professional role in which he would be equipped with negotiation skills. Calley's vision of the peacemaker is one who takes a tribalistic and occult approach to resolving disputes. The other approach that the peacemaker can take is one of conflict resolution. However the peacemaker in the Pentecostal church is unlikely to be trained to use conflict resolution skills and no subordinate can challenge the leader without biblical reasons. Some biblical reasoning, if taken literally, to withdraw, does not encourage healing.

Dr. Gwen Rose

The URC theologians see the word of God present in the church as the source of harmony and order. According to URC minister Godfrey (2002), reformed worshippers such as those in the URC believe the second Helvetic Confession which states "The preaching of the Word of God *is* the Word of God. God is also present and speaks to the people through the sacrament. The minister is called by God through the congregation to lead worship by the authority of his office. The minister speaks the Word of God to the people and speaks the words of the people to God except in instances where the congregation as a whole raises its voice to God in unison." Such a view of the Word can play an equally ambivalent role in dispute resolution as the Pentecostal view of the Spirit.

Stacey (1977) and Gaunton (1997) reinforce the importance of using the variety of gifts given by the Holy Spirit to several members for the common good, especially building the body of Christ. In the Old Testament the Holy Spirit is the Spirit of the Lord, revealing the character and the purpose of God to his people. Isaiah 61:1 alludes to the Holy Spirit with the words: 'The spirit of the Lord God is upon me because the Lord hath anointed me to preach good tidings unto the meek.' One of the symbolic evidence of the gift of the Holy Spirit is narrated in Acts 2 'When the day of Pentecost had fully come, they were all with one accord in one place. Suddenly there came a sound from heaven like a rushing mighty wind and it filled the whole house where they were sitting. This evidence is accepted by both URC and COGIC although the practice of COGIC is more prominent. The demonstration of this evidence is expected from all church members in all the churches. Members who are filled with the Holy Spirit often pray with and for others to be filled or anointed with the Holy Spirit. In the URC the practice of speaking in tongues is not a church wide activity and is practiced only by individual members.

The prosperity gospel tele-evangelists, Kenneth Copeland, and his wife Gloria (Copeland 1990) describes five steps that any believer can take to receive the Holy Spirit: ask without fear, accept that God says you will receive the Holy Spirit, speak no more English, open your mouth wide and drink the Holy Spirit, breathing as deeply as possible, raise your voice and use the lips of your tongue and voice to speak, and finally allow the living waters to flow from you with the greatest freedom. Copeland quotes several passages in Ephesians and John where the gift of the Holy Spirit is promised to all believers and argues that healing belongs to people the moment they are born into God's family. Many mainstream Christians, cited by Oppenheimer (2011), assert there is no evidence that the above practice actually works: there is no scripture to support the practice and they even maintain that this is an occult technique borrowed from Hinduism in which the prana (breathing) energy fills the air. There was no evidence of this practice in the observation of the healing activities in either of the two congregations used for this study.

Although the Holy Spirit was present prior to the day of Pentecost as evidenced in the Old Testament on several occasions such as when Moses selected the elders—, some church members believe that the day of Pentecost is the day that the *power* of the Holy Spirit manifested itself in the community gathered in one place. This community consisted of Jerusalem Jews. Pentecost is the festival which fell on the fiftieth day after the Passover. In modern Christian practice it is the fifth Sunday after Easter Sunday and fifty days after Good Friday. The Book of Acts reports a sound 'as of a mighty wind' and that 'cloven tongues like as of fire' appeared and sat upon each of the men gathered. More impressive was the outburst of *glossolalia*, or speaking in tongues, as the disciples were heard praising God in languages and dialects that differed from their native Galilean Aramaic. The baptism of the Holy Spirit was manifested in this situation and is seen in the church today as the source of the gifts of the Spirit and the gift of healing following Romans 12, which asserts that the gifts of the Holy Spirit are the word of wisdom, word of knowledge, faith, gifts of healing, working of miracles, prophecy, discerning of spirits speaking and interpretation of tongues. This is not dependent on whether members are added to the church or if members leave the church. The gifts are given to the church and the Holy Spirit gives permission to different persons in the church to manifest these gifts (Muddiman 2001). The interview material in section 5.5.2 below shows how this is part of Pentecostal life.

Robbins (1995), however, contends that *glossolalia* is just an innovation by Pentecostalism, the religious movement which began at the turn of the century and is not from God, does not truly honour God, and will not bring people to God. This, Robbins believes, is because the miracles (including Peter healing the sick and lame man) occurring in Acts 2 were intended to occur today but they do not. He argues that *glossolalia* is not a language. The individuals in Acts 2 were heard speaking their own language, meaning the language could be recognized, but according to Robbins (1995) *glossolalia* cannot be recognized as a language. Robbins implies that the manifestation of the Holy Spirit is not always authentic drawing on Acts 8 where Simon Magus offers money to apostles Peter and John, to allow him to lay hands on people so that they can receive the Holy Spirit. In response Peter proclaims: 'Your money perish with you because you thought the gift of God can be purchased.'

A more balanced approach is taken in the article by Richardson and Bowden (1999) in the SCM Dictionary of Christian Theology. They suggest that many theologians conclude from diverse starting points that the self-transcendence of humanity is a genuine experience of the Holy Spirit's 'transcreative power.' They argue that it is clear that, despite cultural variations in practice and theological detail, there is a certain amount of power which is attributed to the Holy Spirit by most ministers, church members, church attendees and those who study theology. The power of the Pastor as described in Ephesians has a limited contribution to spiritual healing; without the power of the Holy Spirit there would be no spiritual healing according to mainstream Christian teaching. Ireland (1997) introduces the gifts of the Holy Spirit using 1 Corinthians 12 'Now about Spiritual gifts, brothers I do not want you to be ignorant.' He further expounds the gifts as 'The word of wisdom, the word of knowledge, faith, healing, prophecy, discerning spirits, tongues and the interpretation of tongues.' The gifts are given to the church and not to an individual. This is internalised in the belief of many church attenders, such as those of the interviewee in the extract below.

Respondent 3 (from the URC) expresses a view of the Holy Spirit as a discerning spirit in action for healing.
'When the healer pray for a person for healing it is good idea especially, it is best if he speak in tongues, first of all to speak quietly in tongues for a minute or two and tell them what you are doing,—'
This extract is repeated in more detail in 5.5. 2

The Holy Spirit as a Gift and Healing as a Gift

The believer is born of God, the source of all regeneration. Respondent 3 refused to believe that spiritual healing can be effected without the power of the Holy Spirit as one of the gifts of faith. He also suggests that healing takes place when the person listens to and hears from God. The respondent implies that miraculous powers are additional to the Power of the Holy Spirit.

Respondent 3 covered topics including belief in healing, belief in the anointing of the Holy Spirit and speaking in tongues. The respondent explained that he has been baptized with the Holy Spirit and has the 'gift' of tongues. He did not relate this to her claim for healing or mention anyone who had administered spiritual healing.

Respondent 3: *Now, gifts of healing do not operate in isolation from other gifts of the Holy Spirit. You will almost certainly need to operate gifts of faith, whilst working the gifts of healing*
This is also stated in 1 Corinthians 12.
If a person, for example have a cancer, which could be terminal, they would need to get the word of God for their situation, they would need to know for certainty in their own heart what God is saying to them, that he will for example, carry them through and the prayers may need to have the same—and you may find that you need gift of miraculous powers to go with that healing as well
You will certainly need to be used by God in the Gifts of the Holy Spirit that has to be with the mind of God. You will need the mind of God's wisdom, to know how and when to pray, the mind of God's Knowledge to know what to pray for and the mind of God's discernment, and knowledge in discernment are vital.

We could conclude that God's wisdom is superior to that of the minister, but then how is this demonstrated in the church where the minister is not operating within the 'mind of God's wisdom?' What happens when the minister does not believe in spiritual healing and members of the congregation have the gift of healing? Coslett (1985) narrates how as a minister he only took tentative steps in the practice of spiritual healing until he had a personal experience. He then wrote "It is my dream that one day Christian churches everywhere will see, accept and use the healing power of Christ as part of everyday ministry." Prior to his personal experience, he too as a minister was doubtful about the power of the Holy Spirit and the gift of healing.

There are many ministers who share similar views because of personal experiences or testimonies from their congregations. As a researcher, I am of the view that there are many ministers whose tentative steps into the ministry of healing will be spurred on by some phenomena, whether personal or ministry related. These experiences will ignite an active interest in the administration of spiritual healing.

Church Governance and Healing: The Minister as a Manager and Healer

The responsibility for spiritual healing in churches lies with the minister as he is legally accountable for the activities of the organization in the same way the Chief Executive or the Director is responsible for the workings of a secular organization. The same legislation applies whether the organization is a commercial venture such as a bank, departmental store, supermarket, or a charitable organization which is not primarily profit making such those funded by the National Health Service or Social Services. In Ephesians 4:11 different skills and gifts (pastors, prophets, apostles, teachers, evangelists, and missionaries) were allocated to the church. This suggests that a range of skills are required in the church in the same way as a range of skills are required in all organizations. Responses to the question about 'who should administer Spiritual healing' elicit responses which always include the minister, although not exclusively.

Respondent 10 (below) has similar views on the pastor's position and the operation of the gift of healing. At the same time these respondents sometimes echo the complaint of Robbins (1995) that many Pentecostal churches ignore the idea that miraculous spiritual gifts may be part of the gifts of the Holy Spirit to ordinary church members as well as to the leaders.

Respondent 10 (COGIC): *That is a good question! (Pause) Obviously we have the Pastor, but not only the Pastor because some people are gifted this way.*

Certain people where that is your calling that is your gift, your ministry. The Pastor may not have that. There are different gifts within the church. If there is someone who show that gift coming out, then obviously if we work with the Pastor (not disrespecting the Pastor) then, obviously it is for the Pastor to make that decision to work with the team, to work with the missionary team, then they can confirm that that person have that gift.

Respondent 2 (URC)
The spiritual evangelical churches are members of (GEAR) Group for Evangelical Renewal who has been trying to encourage a healing ministry since the inception of the URC.
The Concept of Spiritual healing is growing.
Interviewer: How do you promote members with the gift of spiritual healing?
Respondent: The person with the gift of healing can become involved in GEAR or Spring Harvest. There is training for the healing ministry.

In the above extract the respondent clearly states that to be able to administer spiritual healing is a gift. He also implies that the person with this gift is chosen by God and is probably the minister. This person can receive training under the membership of the Group for Evangelical Renewal (GEAR). The blessing of the minister to develop this ministry would probably make for an easier transition into training. However that this may be outside the minister's domain there indicates that there are some aspects of church and the Christian life that reside outside of ministerial control. This respondent implies that there is room for the development of the ministry of spiritual healing in the URC.

Respondent 10 expresses a belief that although the NHS doctors are doing a good job they may well come to a place where they find that they are limited and this is where 'God takes over'.

Interviewer: *How do think the NHS or doctors perceive healing in churches?*
Respondent 10: *I think a lot of them have a great deal of respect for divine healing, some believe that it has its place. Some believe that it has it place and ultimately the medical field is the way forward, some believe that it can actually go hand-in hand. I feel that there is a place for both. God has gifted man anyway to be able to carry out these tests that they do and I would not*

knock them. They do a tremendous job and I also feel that they have their place and when it come to where they can't do anymore then God takes over. There is also the place where I also think that both work hand in hand'

Ministers in COGIC and other black majority churches are expected to participate in healing directly or delegate this as regular activity in the church community. Spiritual healing is physical and psychological. Often black communities have experienced feelings of rejection by the host community and appear find it necessary to seek out spiritual healing amongst their own ministers. They view their ministers as having an understanding of their long social and spiritual journey through generations of slavery, oppression and migration (c.f. Austin-Broos, 1992). These experiences, coupled with their belief in the higher authority and power of God's Holy Spirit leads them to seek prayer for physical, psychological and spiritual healing. They expect the Pastor to facilitate an environment where healing can be instituted. Ministers can do this within and beyond the church environment. When people are confronted with the realities of life threatening situations such as accidents or diagnoses of cancer or mental illness, many patients and their relatives experience a profound challenge to their existing perspective on life and its meaning' (Waldfogel 1997). Where a person may not have attended church for many years, an illness may rekindle their motivation to contact their minister. Sometimes this will be a minister of any denomination in the initial phase followed by a minister from their own denomination. Although they may not have been regular church attendees they may have a sense of faith which has either been dormant or kept alive outside church structures. The illness may be viewed by the individual, the family or the church community as an opportunity to rekindle their spiritual journey and to demonstrate this by resuming regular attendance at church services. When there is a call for prayer these people are usually the first to go forward either for themselves or for their relatives or friends.

Some health professionals are reluctant to admit the element of the 'unknown' in the healing process where there is no physical or physiological explanation as to why or how spiritual healing works. Most doctors take an empirical approach in making use of regimes and drugs, which is not always effective in healing. Gooch (2007) believes that it is not important for nurses to have a religious belief to care for their patients. There is some truth in Gooch's view that nurses do not need religious belief to be effective health care professionals. The fact that they do not believe does not detract from the truth and from the belief of others such as Ewles and Simnett (2003) and other health promoters who tentatively promote the spiritual aspect of healing.

On the other hand, many claims of healing by religious fanatics have resulted in the deaths of vulnerable people who are unable to make decisions and take actions independently. Many of these cases are outlined in Peters (2008) account of healing rituals, children, and the law. Peters (2008:177) claims "Observers from outside the General Assemblies of the Church of the Firstborn, a relatively small Pentecostal church whose roots dates back to the early nineteenth century, claims that its ineffective healing practices has resulted in the deaths of at least two dozen children".

The minister or spiritual healer does not claim to have medical knowledge or to have any knowledge outside of the person seeking healing or their medical practitioner. The interview material shows some people in Black-majority Pentecostal congregations will seek spiritual healing in preference to obtaining a sick note from their doctor, so that they can continue to work. Seeking spiritual healing before going to the doctor for a medical diagnosis means that the person has probably made his own diagnosis and has engaged with the sick role or illness behaviour in a way that is outside of Parsons' (1975) four components of the sick role even if it can fit within some of the later theories of illness behaviour as summarised by Weiss and Lonnquist (2005). The minister or spiritual healer will often advise the person to seek confirmation from their doctor that the condition exists and that the person is not asking for healing for something that is only in their mind. Once they have attended the doctor and have a diagnosis they can then engage with the illness behaviour model. In this situation, as the spiritual healer may encourage the input of the medical doctor if it is impossible for him to claim alternative therapy for the healing process.

For individuals entering Pentecostal worship and healing services, their main purpose may be to seek forgiveness for their sins, spiritual growth and develop a better understanding of God. However, many eventually become aware of the pecking order and ensuing political power struggle within the church. While some choose to close their eyes to these kinds of all-too-human interaction, and focus on personally living a 'godly' life, others complain bitterly about others' promotions and either leave the church or seek promotion elsewhere. Their acceptance of the ideal of the church as led by the Holy Spirit may remain intact, even if they see the operation of their own congregation or church as having failed to live up to that ideal.

Frequently those performing menial tasks are divorced from the management discussions where the allocations of gifts and responsibilities are allocated. Consequently 'working-class' Black majority churches might find it hard to embrace collaborative interaction in the same way as more 'middle-class' congregations with a historic system of congregational government. Black church members were and are still in the minority in the workforce, often engaged in menial, manual and low paid roles, and accustomed not to question management decisions. Within the context of their understanding and their training, the ministers have power and authority as the person who make the final decision in the organization at local and higher organizational level. Pentecostal ministers are not expected to have three years of training for the ministry in the same way as the URC church ministers. Churches such as COGIC train their ministers on the job with minimum book work, a low level of academic study but a high level of commitment to discernment. Their ability to discern is developed through practice over the years and this is largely achieved though the belief in the power and authority of the Holy Spirit.

It is not mandatory for the Pastor to have all of the spiritual gifts. Popular religious writers whose work can be found in the church bookstalls at the front of the churches, such as Meyer (1995) or the constantly evolving Scripture Union "Lifeguide" *Spiritual Gifts* (Hummel and Hummel 1990 Stevens 2004,) emphasise a pastor does not have to have all the gifts of a leader. It is important as with all effective leaders he has the knowledge and skill to delegate and appoint others to positions where they can function to their best for the growth and survival of the organization. Hummel and Hummel (1990) warn that it is imperative that the Pastor understands the purpose of the gifts of prophecy and speaking in tongues so that corporate worship may be conducted in a fitting and ordered manner. Respondent 11 (COGIC) echoes these popular texts:

Interviewer: *The conventional churches, they are very ritualistic in the sense that they would—What I'm thinking is that if someone has the gift of healing, because the church is ritualistic in their approach to healing, the person who is gifted may not get the opportunity to practise because the church's approach to healing is ritualistic*
Respondent 11 . . . : *That is also wrong. In our church the minister encourages everybody to take part in what is going on, so if you are interested in the healing ministry, come we will help you. Some people feel. 'Oh I can't do this or I that'. So anyone of you can do it because it is not you, it is the Holy Spirit who is going to do it, so it is your faith and you being able to listen to God, because everybody that the Holy Spirit uses they are able to listen they know the prompting of the Holy Spirit. Those with the gift of healing, they see and they feel. It is not everybody they see that they lay hands on. It depends on where the Holy Spirit leads them. It is time we get out of the rituals in the church and allow the Holy Spirit to work.*

Rosato (1999) argues that the "prompting of the Holy Spirit" denotes supernatural power that cannot be given by man. However this can only be exercised in the church community by the permission of the minister or a body of ministers. Although there is a concept of supernatural application of power, similar restrictions to those in any organization are in operation.

In a similar vein respondent 2 states '*the chosen person becomes a front line target and needs nurturing and close monitoring*' indicating that although there may be a supernatural gift for healing, it is necessary for this gift to operate under close monitoring and cannot be used unsupervised. '*There is no discipleship*' implies that the Holy Spirit cannot be disciplined in the same way that that a Christian or an employee is disciplined by the church or the employer.

Selecting Spiritual Leaders in the Christian Churches

There is much popular religious literature aimed at potential church leaders who have not yet received theological training, advising them on the qualities to look for in themselves and others. Many skilled leaders according to Winston (2002) do not believe that they are called to become leaders when they become members of a church. They expect to be led by the Holy Spirit or some other force outside human skills. To some extent this is true, although leadership skills are part of the character of the person who is selected to lead. One of the tasks of the Holy Spirit in action through selected individuals is to call godly leaders in the kingdom. Winston is echoed by other writers as diverse as the liberal Presbyterian male feminist Daniel Patte (1995), the Catholic editors of the *Jerome Bible commentary* (Brown et al 1996), the *Cambridge Companion to Biblical Interpretation*, (Barton 1998), as well as the URC divine McGrath (1997), who all assert leaders experiences different kinds of calling in different ways. The calling of Moses, Samuel and David are cited as examples of leaders being called and selected by the Holy Spirit.

In respect of questions on which Pentecostals, like other denominations tends to be divided, is the question of women in ministry. According to Barton (1998) the interpretation of biblical texts is always through the eyes of the age in which they are read. Women in leadership positions within the Old Testament are few and it is illustrated in many biblical texts such as when Moses was instructed to select seven elders who were male. The outline of how women should dress and conduct themselves in a worship service is directed to women from the culture of the author who wrote the book of Timothy and Corinthians. Women from western culture may now think they do not have to abide by the same rules and the challenge to male power has permeated to other sections of women's lives especially in the work place and public organizations. In Toulis' (1997) chapter on 'Wives, mothers and female saints', she argues that the gender processes in the New Testament Church of God (which has similarities to COGIC) 'are broadly comparable with other Protestant traditions'.

Tutu's (1986) advocacy of a politically active church in his book '*Crying in the Wilderness*' encouraged many Black churches to view their leaders as people who should actively engage with the wider community and politics. Many in mainstream churches accept the view, however, that the churches should not interfere in politics. However much church leaders are given apparent high regard, they are still viewed with disdain by many sections of society. It also so happens that the leaders that Tutu refers to, like the COGIC leaders discussed by Thomas-Juggan (2000), are all men. Women's ministry, where it occurs, is seen as a kind of exception to the rule.

Many churches will not ordain women as ministers and this continues to be controversial subject. In COGIC women are not ordained as elders or pastors, but they are ordained as missionaries, evangelists and deacons. The titles are not easily explainable nor do they have a clear rationale. Women normally do not serve the Lord's Supper. As in all other sections of society women take responsibility for the daily organizational activities partly because they are in a majority. There are appointed persons who can invite speakers outside the church to preach, teach and heal. A recommendation must first go to the Pastor who has the authority to make a decision to take the recommendation to the church committee. These appointed persons may also have the authority to decide on matters relating to the Missionary Sunday, the day when the missionaries (ladies) conduct the service or the Youth Sunday, the day when the youth leader conduct the service. These are on a set day in the month, such as the first Sunday or third Sunday.

Allowing women ministers in URC to serve Communion is left to the decision of the local leadership as there is no clause in the policy for the ordination of ministers (URC General Assembly, 1982) that excludes women. Women, though still in a minority, represent the church at all levels of the organisational functions and duties. These include wider church meetings such as Regional Church Council, Synod, Mission Council or General Assembly. Councils meet quarterly, Synods meet twice yearly and the General Assembly meets annually.

The church as an organization and the church as part of the community, part of society, is the subject of multiple expectations regarding leadership. Spiritual Leaders historically and spiritual leaders today rely on a theological context in which to live, work and make decisions. They accept that there are eternal parameters for temporal decision making, but they are also required to comply with the corporate policies of the organization and also legal policies and to enable others to do the same. There are some similarities in the use of wisdom and skills of the spiritual leader and the use of wisdom and professional judgement of the health care professionals. There are also differences in that the healthcare professionals have the added knowledge of the homeostatic operations of the human body, but have to rely on wisdom in the use of this knowledge. The spiritual leader relies primarily on the wisdom and guidance of the spirit and the experiences of delivering healing.

The Pastor of COGIC is chosen and trained through a long process (up to seven years) of apprenticeship and a demonstration of life commitment of service to God and the people. This training does not always include paper qualifications. The URC minister is trained for a minimum of three years and allocated to a church as an apprentice, followed by salaried employment within the organization. Some ministers in the URC are trained in the same way as a paid minister but appointed as non-stipendiary. The main difference is that not all COGIC ministers go through a formal academic training program. The older ministers are may demonstrate the skills of leadership in practice but not on paper.

The view within both congregations tends to follow the mainstream view outlined by Clebsch and Jaekle (1983) that the four main areas of pastoral function are healing, sustaining, guiding and reconciling. Ministers with a vocational call are expected to have personal qualities such as the ability to heal, discern, heal, counsel and generally care for people. These qualities, however, are not limited to church ministers. It is a requirement of human survival to have the ability to care for others. Some will care more than others and many people have responsibility for care that resembles pastoral care in their day to day occupation, be this paid or voluntary work. Others such as nurses, doctors, human resource managers have this as part of their paid employment. The minister is responsible for delegating his role and function to appropriately appointed persons as elders, deacons, evangelists, prayer leaders and missionaries.

The picture painted by Clebsch and Jaekle (1983) of the main areas of pastoral function have similarities to secular discussions of professional functions that encourage and support people to develop intellectually and emotionally in the caring organizations such as teaching, nursing traditional and complementary medicine and social work. In all these areas there is a focus on relationship with self and others on a physical, emotional and spiritual level. Anbu (2008) relates the terms emotional and social intelligence, which were brought to wide public attention by the pop psychologist Coleman (2006) to nurses as they function in their every day duties of caring for the sick as care practitioner, manager or both. Coleman (2006) classifies the emotional intelligence as self awareness, self regulation and self motivation and the social intelligence as social awareness, empathy and social skills. Empathy crosses over the boundaries of the emotional and the social and the person using the skills of empathy develops the ability (of the healer) to be protected against becoming ill with the condition of the person who is being healed.

The pastor/minister is also expected to have a well developed emotional intelligence, emotional maturity and social intelligence to be an effective church leader. The spiritual healer who may be visiting minister or a church member is also expected to function at a high emotional intelligence level and requires a leader who has a similar level of awareness and functioning. The leader does not necessarily have to have the same level of development of the gift of healing as this is given to the church rather than to individuals. He is expected to know when to accept the leading of the Holy Spirit.

Where there is no revelation, the people cast off restraints according to Proverbs 29:18. A possible interpretation of this verse is that where there is no spiritual inspiration there is likely to be chaos. All organization is dependent on good leadership and vision to survive and the church is no different. Without effective leadership the organization and its purpose is likely to collapse and eventually become fruitless. A care management textbook (Rogers and Reynolds 2003) is as likely as any popular religious book to insist the leader must be able to motivate people to 'catch the vision'. Many organizations have 'mission statements' and 'visions'. These uses of biblical terminology are often used in non-church organizations without the recognition of their origins. Individual vision must be in tandem with the vision of the wider church and its doctrine, although local authority or NHS care managers are unlikely to be told by their superiors to engage in fasting and prayer, bible studies, witness and visitation of the Holy Spirit like Pentecostal pastors.

Members with the Gift of Healing

Members with the gift of healing, like everyone else, go through a phase of physical, psychological and spiritual development. The extract below from a URC church member who practises healing illustrates the qualities of someone using the gift of healing. Although he is not a leading minister in his church, he is accepted as a minister with the gift of healing as he is also requested and given permission by his minister to deliver healing seminars and healing services in other churches. His participation in the interview came across as though he was presenting a seminar on Spiritual Healing.

Respondent 3: *'When the healer prays for a person for healing it is good idea especially, it is best if he speak in tongues, first of all to speak quietly in tongues for a minute or two and tell them what you are doing, cause you are tuning into the Lord, then by all means pray for what they ask for, but he may find that God puts a question in your mind to ask them, or a realization that there is something else he should be praying for as well as what they ask, then have a conversation with the person about what God has laid on his mind. The healer will often be astonished to find that what he finishes up praying for is different to what they ask for and get a better result. It may not give them the healing they ask for at that time, but it will give them something better and the healing will come to them later This is the gift of knowledge, knowing God's mind and what should be prayed for and you will certainly need the gift of discerning the Spirit.*
In the scriptures you will see that on two occasions Jesus healed men who were deaf and dumb; on one of the occasion he did so by casting out the spirit and on one occasion he did so by ministering physical healing. If the healer try and cast out the spirit from somebody when they need physical healing, the healer can traumatize them. If on the other hand you try and administer physical healing when there is demonic force at work, healing will not take place and the demon will be quietly laughing. The healer has to know what he is praying for. Another thing that is needed with the knowledge of discernment is that when praying for somebody, for Christian healing, for Jesus to heal them, there will be occasions when it is right to lay hands on them and there will be occasions when it will be right to give a command. If the certainty comes on you to give a command, then give a command and when you do so do it with authority.
For example, when praying for cancer victims it is perfectly valid if the Lord lays it on you to command the cancer to 'DIE' in the Name of Jesus and to 'condemn' in the Name of Jesus. The implication is that the cancer is some form of demonic force and you would be amazed how often it works, but you must know from the Lord whether that is the way to pray or not. This is gift of healing working with all the other gifts of the Holy Spirit.'

This speaker may approve of speaking in tongues, but his views on members with the discerning power of the Spirit are not so far from those of the liberal theologian Moltman (1997:19) who wrote: "Where Jesus is, there is life, sick people are healed, sad people are comforted and the demonic spirits are driven out". Like Carr (1989), he sees the healer, not necessarily the minister, as a window through which the transaction of healing takes place in two directions. (God and the healer, on one side and the person seeking healing on the other side).

Spiritual healers in the observed congregations are not allowed to accept financial reward for administering healing during services. This situates the relationship between patient and healer outside of the material exchange of conventional medical practitioners.

Becoming a Member and Learning to Heal

Membership of both churches is to a large extent under the power and control of the minister, although recommendations for membership come from other sources such as infant baptism and other ministers. The process of becoming a member in COGIC and URC is outlined in section 4.11. Transfer of membership from another church within each organization uses broadly the same mechanisms for adults with established membership. All members in both Churches are allowed to participate in the healing service by extending their arm towards the person receiving healing although there are specific people who are regarded as healing ministers. The healing minister may not be the same person as the Pastor/Minister.

The healer, not necessarily the minister is a window through which the transaction of healing takes place in two directions. (God, the healer on one side and the person seeking healing on the other side). The transaction operates like black and white, worker and boss, men and women as Carr (1989) explains. The overlap can probably be explained by a psychoanalytical approach, but only those with an understanding of the operation of the Holy Spirit (Carr 1989). The process of learning to heal is synoptic with receiving the gift of healing and the gift of the Holy Spirit as well as practicing these gifts. The style of worship in the Pentecostal Church (COGIC) where the 'minister' facilitates the activity of healing, encourages the practice of healing through atonement and forgiveness of sin.

Conclusion

This chapter has discussed the way in which the theology of the spirit legitimates the spiritual healing practices of the two congregations observed. These beliefs and practices mean that the state of health of those seeking spiritual healing is to some extent under the power of leaders. Within these congregations, by and large the leaders take a holistic view of health. Health for them is not merely a state of biological (homeostasis) balance; it is also a spiritual state. Therefore, the ministers believe firmly in a place of spirituality for the healer and for the church as an organization. Christian tradition understands the work of the Spirit in three broad areas of revelation, salvation and Christian life. The classic Pentecostal churches see the Holy Spirit as the link between healing and salvation as the agency by which Christ's atoning death brings healing from sickness and disease. Historic Protestantism regards salvation as the healing of human life, which emboldens us to pray for physical healing, which may, as in Jesus' lifetime, be granted. Both, however, think of worship, prayer, the laying on of hands and church music as much or more as health promotion activities and the relief of suffering than as 'cures' in the clinical sense. The next chapters look first at suffering and its relief, and then at prayer, the laying on of hands, and considers the role of music.

Chapter Three

Suffering and Healing

Introduction

This chapter presents analysis evidence about perceptions of suffering and the process of exercising faith in seeking spiritual healing. It relates the data from the observations and interviews to the literatures, whether medical, biblical or in popular culture. There is also an exploration of suffering as psychological or physical pain and homeostatic imbalance as outlined in Chapter Two. A person who is suffering is identified as one with a physical, emotional or mental imbalance which could be short term or long term. This description fits all the respondents and all those who volunteered to have spiritual healing administered to them during healing services in the URC and the invitation for prayer in COGIC. In any one human experience there may be mixture of more than one element of suffering where the person is subjected to pain, defeat or change.

Suffering in Context

Religious ideas are a prime source of concepts for coping with suffering. Each person and probably each church have a different perception of suffering and the cultural background of the people may have some influence on this view. Daya (2005) suggests that although religions vary, they offer some common responses to common experience of all humans regardless of their cultural, racial or religious background, going on to suggest the Buddhist psychology embodied in the "four noble truths" presents a template for thought about symptoms, diagnosis, prognosis and treatment for human suffering.

Nonetheless, human thought systems present a wide variety of ways of theorising suffering and pain (sometimes used interchangeably as both are about a person's physical mental and emotional (or affective) response to pain at different levels of intensity). Though human suffering has been prioritised during much of history, for some people suffering relates to all living things including animals and plants. In the thought of non-religious philosophers such as Bentham, (2001, originally 1859) on utilitarian principle, Popper (2002) on interpretation, and Katz (1990) on scientific knowledge, there is the idea of promoting the greatest good or happiness for the greatest number of people. This is proposed to be achieved by balancing the reduction of suffering with the enhancement of happiness and can be seen to draw on the same array of concepts as previous religious thought. Traditional religious discussions of the suffering of Christ do show, in a way, its utility, as Swenson (2005:44) postulates that 'Jesus suffers with us'. McGrath's (1995) discussion on the Doctrine of God suggests Christ, as the representative of God in the flesh, experiences suffering as a result of making people in his image and experiencing their pain. Although suffering is subject to cultural interpretations, for a person to experience such extreme pain as was depicted in the crucifixion of Christ raises the similar universal questions. One cultural interpretation of suffering is proposed by Warrington (2008) who suggests that the concept of suffering is neglected by Pentecostals who move too quickly to the victory and glory associated with the result of overcoming suffering, strength through weakness, light through darkness and salvation through the death and resurrection of Jesus. In seeking healing and liberation from suffering through salvation Black church members aim to heal 'the brokenness of black existence' which MacRobert (1988) suggests as the context out of which Pentecostalism emerged.

Myss (1997) exemplifies how popular self-help writing brings together medical, theological and utilitarian ideas in its detailed exploration of the interconnectedness of the mind body and spirit implies that if the body suffers then so do the mind and the spirit. We can hear echoes of them all in the thoughts on suffering expressed by Respondent 4 below, and they are not necessarily consistent with each other as the respondent addresses different situations. The respondent is unsure of her views on suffering as she narrates her views of her sister's experience and the experiences of parents who have lost a child. She believes that parents who have lost a child suffer but her sister is not suffering as her sister has found a way of coping. The practical conceptualisation of suffering relates of course to the context in which it is experienced. It is different in hospital to what it is in the home. As the philosopher Cowley (2009) points out "Consider the hospital: in no other single building in human society is there such an overwhelming concentration of suffering, despair and death" except perhaps, he admits in a footnote, prison. Mere philosophers lack the authority to tell doctors what to do, but he asserts, "On the other hand, by far the most sophisticated accounts of the *meaning* of suffering and death have been offered by the major world religions" and argues theologians do tackle the doctors' dilemmas. Many people in hospital look to their religious leaders and their religious institutions for some relief of their suffering and the NHS professionals can also learn from them. From a nursing perspective, Johnson (2008) echoes Cowley in suggesting that religious professionals can help nurture the compassion for the suffering of others that should characterise professionals such as nurses during their training.

Personal suffering is related to the person's relationship with God and can be perceived as covert or overt pain. In Jaye's (2001) comparison of Pentecostal and secular General Practitioners, it was found that healing and suffering was viewed as a complex process by Pentecostals going beyond a purely curative approach, because Pentecostals explained suffering using a Christian as well as a medical framework. In Jaye's study, a secular view of curing indicates a narrow focus on the efficiency of treatment and in some situations suffering in human understanding can only end with the end of life, the process of bereavement on which the literature was examined in Chapter Two.

The understandings of suffering considered in this chapter show a need for healing from a sense of rejection, as well as from disease, which is an indication of how suffering has spiritual, emotional and social as well as physical aspects. In comparing this to the healing of a physical wound, healing by first intention is not applicable as there is no obvious wound or obvious operation except for bereavement or a situation such as loss of employment. Spiritual healing therefore is healing by second intention where the wound is open or gaping (c.f. Waugh et al. 2006) and healing takes place from the deeper tissues/psychological state, although this may not be recognized by the respondent or be seen by the healer.

The contributors to Lucas (1997) list some situations which inevitably result in suffering addressed by Christian healing. Some of these are diseases or sicknesses of all kinds, especially long term incurable and painful conditions. A physical illness such as a gastric ulcer or breast cancer can be treated with medication or possibly surgery. If the cause of the ulcer is due to lifestyle, personality or is genetic, medication and or surgery will treat the effect and not the cause. Healing the underlying cause is something different and more profound.

Holmes and Rahe (1967) go one step further to develop a social-psychological readjustment scale which presents a table of ailments that can cause stress and probably depression and ill health in an individual. They give each a score in order of intensity of suffering. Most of these situations are not physical illnesses but the psychological effect of the illness such as loss of lifestyle and the process required to adjust to a different lifestyle.

Superficial healing will not address the suffering, as suffering requires a deeper approach to healing. Most theologians, both the academic ones discussed in section 2.4, and the popular ones cited in this chapter, insist that healing and relieving suffering requires a more holistic approach where the wholesomeness of God is operational. Holistic care is where the person experiences a touch of love and comfort and not just the release of pain. The concept of hospice care embraces the relief of suffering and the best quality of life for those who are dying and not just the relief of pain.

Perceptions of Suffering

Each church has a different perception on suffering and the cultural background of the people influences this. The URC think that suffering can bring about a kind of epiphany is shedding light or developing wisdom on issues which defy understanding (c.f. Jones 1980). An increased understanding of imbalance by the healer and the person seeking healing can relieve suffering. The suffering of the people from COGIC could be viewed as illuminated by the historical memories of slavery which is not the same for majority of church attendees to the URC (c.f. Austin-Broos

1992). Developing a better understanding of issues can reduce the suffering (pain) caused by a particular situation or incidence. However suffering and healing, as perceived by members of both churches, is experienced regardless of their class or occupational status. The need for health promotion and healing activities also cuts across class.

The ambiguities of respondents' understandings of suffering are exemplified in the response from respondent 4 (URC) quoted below. This respondent was asked directly about views on suffering and indicated that her understanding of suffering is not clear.

Interviewer: *What do you think about suffering?*
Respondent: *Well—I don't think I've resolved feelings about suffering. There are many people who suffer—Young people who died or—someone who has, from breast cancer. I think she suffered and J who has had a major operation to remove a tumour from behind her eye. She is now looking well, but I think she suffered a lot this was about a year ago. J who is not well herself has had to care for her—I don't know what the prognosis is going to be but he does not think that he has cancer. He got lots of other things, How much suffering should you have? That, I really can't understand that; I really can't understand that.*
Interviewer: *It is possible that we get as much as we can handle.*
Respondent: *Some people say that but I don't know.*
Interviewer: *We can't make that decision*
Respondent:Llots of people go through life without much suffering.
Interviewer: *(surprised!) Do you think so?*
Respondent: *with an adamant YES! I have a sister—*
[She—proceeded to describe the sister's ailments in details. Her sister is selfish etc and does not do anywhere as much as she should do for her husband who has to go into hospital. It is very sad, very sad because one daughter has to stop work for days to help to look after her father.
She will get home help—and she will do but it takes away an afternoon that she could use for something else.]
Interviewer: *Do you think some of that is suffering?*
Respondent: *Not for my sister she has always managed to get everyone doing things for her throughout her life. She has never actually done very much for herself or anyone else.*

This respondent's perception and understanding of suffering is unclear. She acknowledges suffering as physical pain, yet although her sister complains of a physical illness, this is regarded as malingering, in the sense of Asher (2002) and a means of avoiding caring for another person. The respondent views the parents of a child or a young person who dies or someone who has breast cancer as suffering, yet her sister, who has many illnesses, does not appear to have that right to suffer. It is possible that this respondent is suffering for her family and her way of dealing with her denial or misunderstanding of suffering is to project this onto her sister as not suffering.

One person can share another person's suffering by empathizing with them, because they have experienced a similar situation or are actually sharing the situation with them. The suffering of one family member radiates to other family members in varying degrees; yet this does not appear to be happening in this scenario.

This respondent has unresolved feelings about suffering; her views expressed these feelings in more than one way. She describes sufferers as those with a physical condition such as a heart condition in a young person or someone with breast cancer whilst also mentioning 'the parents of young people who die.' The respondent gave an example of someone who has suffered but is now 'looking well' but also acknowledged that this person will continue to suffer as there are other physical ailments.

She also thinks that not everyone suffers and although her sister has lots of ailments, she is selfish as her sister does not do enough for her husband who is ill and has to go into hospital. When asked if her sister was suffering she said that her sister was not suffering because her sister has always managed to get other people to do things for her and has not done much for herself throughout her life. She implied that her sister was a malingerer as described by Asher (2002) who described self-manufactured illnesses.

In her account of suffering this respondent perceived other people's illness as suffering but she could not perceive her sister's suffering. It may be that there is a superimposition of her own experiences onto that of her sister as she is so emotionally close to her sister.

Respondent 4 gives as an example of suffering when a young person dies, without specifying if this meant that that person is suffering in death or the suffered before death or their loved ones left behind are suffering. This concept of suffering may depend on the belief of a life after death where there is change and we imagine that the change could be a life of continued suffering or relief from the suffering. The fact that death causes suffering at different levels for those who are alive cannot be disputed. When a young person dies it causes suffering because of the loss of financial and other contribution that that person could make to society had they lived? It appears to be a wasted life. Psychological suffering can be as real as physical suffering and the two cannot be separated into discrete aspects of the person.

Respondent 4's somewhat judgmental approach to her sister may mirror traditional Christian interpretations of the suffering of Job, the biblical character who is taken to illustrate the suffering of the innocent in her comments on children and the parents of children who die. C.S. Lewis (2003) argued that the ultimate purpose of suffering is for man to repent and return to the creator in humility in the same way that Job repented and was healed of his suffering. A moral contrast is offered between those who accept suffering patiently in this way, such as the woman who had lived with the issue of blood for more than thirty years whom Jesus healed. She did not want to continue in her state of suffering and believed that she could be healed and she was healed. This can be contrasted with the man at the Gate Beautiful (Acts 3) who had suffered from birth, but had accepted his suffering and was not seeking to be healed. He was seeking a way to continue in his way of living by begging alms.

Respondent 4's account of suffering suggests that only physical conditions such as an obvious physical disability *are* suffering rather than just one cause of suffering, hence her views that her sister was not suffering although she complained of many less-than-disabling physical ailments. Maybe she was unable to feel for her sister as this could cause psychological suffering for her (the respondent). Her sister had also distanced herself from her by not communicating with her. Consequently she (the respondent) focused her sympathy on her sister's daughter and her sister's husband. Her accounts of suffering confirm her statement, '*I have mixed feelings about suffering*'. This may be true for many people.

Respondent 10 (COGIC) was aware that she herself was ill and suffering. She was seeking spiritual healing through her own prayers and when her own prayers were not effective she sought the assistance of the minister. She believed that she was directed to go to the meeting and there she would be healed (the first part of her story). The second part of her story illustrates her denial of her own suffering and whilst seeking healing for her sister whom she believed was more in need of prayer at that time. The healer probably surmised something was wrong and probably linked this with the pregnancy because this was the most obvious sign that he could see.

Respondent 10

'I was ill for about 10 weeks and had two courses of antibiotics. After the second course, my voice had still not returned. There was a meeting at headquarters for the church and I heard a voice said to me go to the meeting. I went to the meeting.

During the message the preacher said 'your healing is in you coming today' I felt that these words were God speaking to me directly and at the invitation for prayer I went forward for prayer. This is not something that I do lightly or on a regular basis. As I stood at the altar, I started to pray and I was playing with my throat, like this! using my hands to gently touch and rub my throat.' (as she said this she was demonstrating her actions during her prayer)

'I felt that something had moved in my throat but I did not say anything to anyone.

On the Sunday following this I went to church and there was only one member of the praise and worship team. This was not an experienced member and I felt that I really could not leave her to sing alone. So I prayed and joined her. As I started to sing the voice was not coming through. I was so scared, my throat was dry and I found it difficult to swallow as it was more than ten weeks that I was unable to sing. However I continued to try singing and gradually I started to sing and sing. I was truly blessed and was able to bless the congregation on that day.

This period of time allowed me to humble myself and be a part of the congregation but I really did miss this aspect of worship for myself.

The second experience that I can remember was when I was carrying my fifth son. The doctor told me that I had a clot on my lung and I had to go to hospital every day for anti-clotting treatment. After the treatment, the doctor told me that my baby was not growing and he was very small. I did not tell my husband this; I kept it to myself.

One Sunday there was visiting preacher and I went for prayer for my sister who was in hospital. As I stood at the altar, the minister came to me and said 'is there some thing wrong with your pregnancy/baby?' I said 'Everything is fine.' He had been making eye contact with me during the service although I did not know him.

He went around the other people at the altar, and came back to me and said 'what is wrong with your baby?' I could not hold back any longer so I said 'Yes something is wrong but my husband does not know.' Here I was being more concerned about my husband than I was about my baby. He called my husband from the church office and asked me the same question in front of him and prayed with us. He told me to talk to my baby, to tell the child that I love him and generally talk to him. When my son was born he was the size of my other children at birth. The stunted growth in my womb was corrected.

This respondent demonstrated some level of faith in her own prayers and the prayers of the minister by praying for herself and then going to the altar. It appears that she experienced some suffering relating to her pregnancy and tried to deny this by seeking prayer for her sister who was in hospital with a more obvious illness.

Suffering and Faith

Lewis (2003) postulates that a 'rational' faith can fall to pieces when it is confronted with suffering as a personal reality rather than a mild theoretical disturbance.' However, the respondents show that for them faith and suffering are inextricably linked and that the extent of faith in a belief system can minimize the severity of suffering although this severity is subjective and can only be measured by the person who is experiencing the phenomena of suffering. Faith is intricately linked with suffering as both are invisible human experiences which are also linked with healing and spirituality in some form within all cultures.

Faith is a theological concept where there is acceptance of over-arching truth without empirical proof (c.f. Stacey 1977, Gaunton 1997), as the author of Hebrews 11 puts it 'the substance of things hoped for, and the evidence of things not seen.' Such faith is not always religious. Although faith and religious beliefs are closely linked, it is possible that a person who has doubts about his religious beliefs may have faith in some things such as herbal medicine (Stacey 1977). The experience of an illness, suffering and pain or disease is also inextricably linked by respondents with faith. Christianity has clear statements of faith in the format of creeds which guide the majority of denominations and their belief. Credally-based Christian denominations claim that truth is truth and practise this truth within the principles of orthodoxy, some developed relatively early in the development of the church (Young 1993). This is illustrated in the comment from respondent 2 and in the statement on the nature of faith below.

Respondent 2 (URC)
Gifts of healing do not operate in isolation from other gifts of the Holy Spirit. The healer will almost certainly need to operate **gifts of faith**, *whilst working the gifts of healing. This is also stated in 1 Corinthians 12. If a person, for example, have a cancer, which could be terminal, they would need to get the word of God for their situation. They would need to know for certainty in their own heart what God is saying to them, that He will for example, carry them through and the prayers may need to have the same—and you may find that the gift of miraculous powers go with that healing as well. The healer will certainly need to be used by God in the Gifts of the Holy Spirit that has to be with the mind of God. You will need the mind of God's wisdom, to know how and when to pray, the mind of God's knowledge to know what to pray for and the mind of God's discernment and knowledge in discernment are vital.*

This is broadly in accordance with the statement of the United Reform Church (2008) on the Nature, Faith and Order of the URC:

'With the whole Christian church, the URC believes in one God, Father, son and Holy Spirit., The living God, the only God ever to be praised. The life of faith to which we are called is the spirit's gift continually received through the Word of the Sacraments and for Christian life together. We acknowledge the gifts and answer the call giving thanks for the means of grace.'

The highest authority for what we believe and do is God's word in the Bible alive for the people today through the help of the spirit. We respond to this Word, whose servants we are with God's people through the years. We accept with thanksgiving to God, the witness to the Catholic faith in the 'Apostles' and the Nicene creeds. We acknowledge the declarations made in our own traditions by Congregationalists, Presbyterians and Church of Christ in which they stated the faith and sought to make its implications clear. Faith alive and active gift of an eternal source renewed for every generation. We conduct our life according to the basis of union in which we give expression of our faith in forms which we believe contains the essential elements of the Christ's life both catholic and reformed.'

This statement does not mention suffering explicitly; however it should be remembered, as stated before that faith and suffering is inextricably linked. The statement is an adaptation of the definition of faith of the Council of Chalcedon (Gaunton 1997) and sets out the URC belief in faith, the gift of Holy Spirit, the Sacraments for Christian life. COGIC uses almost the same statement of Faith for those who come into membership by transfer or baptism. During baptism classes the statement is used by both churches but members may not revisit the statement unless they are present when new members are received into the church. The statement of faith makes no direct reference to healing although there is reference to the gift of the spirit. If the gift of the Spirit includes the gift of healing, then it is inherent that the statement of faith is also a statement on healing and suffering. Their statement of faith underpins the belief of each congregation in the way they practise spiritual healing and is explored in more depth by members from both churches who undertake courses to increase their understanding of the Christian doctrine.

The extract below, from respondent 2, comments on the use of passive and active faith, the gift of faith and a belief in the distinction between having faith or not having faith. This respondent compartmentalizes faith and healing *'gifts of healing I will come to in a moment'*, for the purpose of clarity although the issues of faith and healing are closely interlinked. Faith is being promoted as evidenced even when the evidence is not obvious.

The message of knowledge, not the knowledge of man's learning but the knowledge of God, which knows what to pray for the person at that time.

the gift of faith, not the faith of salvation, but a sudden certainty in the circumstance and knowing what is being asked for will be actually given, and also receiving a word for that person during the illness which may carry them through that illness.

Gifts of healing, I will come to in a moment.

What I teach on this matter is, that you should never dump on people that they do not have faith and neither should you dump on yourself that you don't have faith. You should get on with praying for them.

Now in Romans 12, Paul tells the Christian to make a sober judgment of themselves based on the amount of faith that they have. One of the things that this means is the amount of power within them and if you study carefully the way the gifts of miraculous powers are operated you will find that there is a relationship between power and what resides in the person's body.

Healing, where there is no direct spiritual approach usually involves some kind of faith approach where the person seeking healing has faith in the medication or the health professional's ability to help them towards recovery from perceived suffering.

Faith-healing is heavily criticized by some non-believers and some believers, whilst advocating their own religious healing, criticize that of other faith practices as superstitious and idolatrous. This makes it difficult to position healing and suffering in the context of faith. Most believers also hold that there are undoubtedly false teachings on faith healing and this may vary in severity from group to group and from individual to individual. Many people attribute sickness to demonic forces and rely on activities such as exorcism as a tool of faith healing. Others blame sickness on failure to believe or on sin and others make claims as healers for financial reward, which is criticised as throughout Jesus' life on earth in the flesh there was never any recording of a request for financial contribution for the healing work that He did and what He taught his disciples. Understanding these critiques from within, and the way in which criteria of authenticity or acceptability were established is crucial to co-operation with faith communities.

Respondent: *I argue with my doctors a lot*
Interviewer: *Let's take it away from you! Do you think that if the doctor is giving someone medicine to take they should take it?*

Health Promotion—Spiritual Healing

Respondent*: I can't tell anyone what to take and what not to take. It depends on what they believe. If I say don't take something and you don't believe what good will that do? I cant tell anyone—not even my son, being my own child—When he was young I could decide and I could pray because he could not make a choice but once he can make a choice everybody has the right to make a choice, it is their right. No one has the right to choose for another person, so even if I say don't take it and you are doubting it is not going to do any good because your mind is somewhere else, so it is faith. I believe that God can heal me and that is why I am healed.*

The question did not include faith although it was the intention of the researcher to ascertain the respondent's view on faith and suffering. The respondent made it quite clear that it was up to the individual whether they had faith in the medicine/treatment offered by their doctor will relieve their suffering As a spiritual healer she had no authority over the individual. She illustrated this further by using he role as a parent in making decision for children under a certain age but when the child reach a certain age the parent has no further authority over what the child does especially in relation to taking medicines. She also explained her own faith in the doctors and the role that prayer plays in her healing. She also states clearly that faith and belief are superimposed on each other.

'So it is faith*. I believe that God can heal me and that is why I am healed.'*

The bible does not condemn, forbid or discourage the use of medicines or proper medical care. In Luke's Gospel Luke was a doctor before he became an apostle and Paul advised Timothy to use some wine to for his stomach problems (1Timothy 5. Although this is a diversion from the rest of the chapter according to Brown et al. (1996), it indicates that the physical health is as important as spiritual and social health. Paul does not suggest that Timothy's illness is caused by a lack of faith; instead Paul suggests that Timothy is seen as a spiritual leader and as a good example. Therefore using faith towards a relief of suffering and healing is not only about using prayer as a tool for healing it could be about using other tools such as a variety of medicines, surgery, herbal medicines, complementary therapies and a good diet. Selected aspects of these methods may assist the body to heal itself of the suffering caused by different ailments and for different people. Faith and suffering are also inextricably linked to illness and disease, matters discussed in the next section.

The Difference between Illness and Disease as Suffering

The account of the respondents illustrates the acceptance of this distinction in society. The acceptance of illness as evidence of a disease licences adopting the sick role. This can be regarded as evidence of real suffering by the sufferer, their family or the wider society. However, often the bio-psycho-social aspect of an illness is determined by the society affected. People can be ill without having a disease and people can have a disease without being ill, although the two are often interlinked. Both facets are culturally determined as outlined in the health behaviour models reviewed by Kasl and Kolb (1996), and Dingwall's (1976) illness action model.

For example the AIDS epidemic has an international as well as a local response. In societies where there is no treatment or people cannot afford medical care, a diagnosis is a death sentence. Before a diagnosis or a label is given to the person who feels ill, death is not imminent; they may refuse to consult with a health professional for fear of being told they have HIV/AIDS. When they do seek medical assistance and have a name to their illness (death sentence) only the immediate family is allowed to know at the discretion of the sufferer and their doctor. HIV/AIDS is one such condition where people can have the disease without feeling ill for a very long time.

In my professional experience there are many people who claim to be ill as an attention seeking exercise. For example when I worked in a children's ward there was a young girl who claimed to be constantly in pain, although she was given all the available painkillers, the pain persisted. Her parents shouted at the doctors and nurses to do something to help their daughter. When I spent some time talking to the child, she revealed that she complained of pain to get her mother's attention as her mother often ignored her. Although she had a disease and was in some pain, she used this to compound her illness and to seek attention from her mother. Mothers who are under a lot of pressure sometimes complain of headache (migraine) so that they can opt out of their responsibilities, which they are then allowed to do, as well as getting sympathy from the family. Without a physical condition that can be treated by a health professional, they would not be regarded as suffering and adopt the sick role as conceptualised by Parsons (1975).

People with diseases such as Alzheimer's, HIV and AIDS, Cancer, though clearly suffering, may choose to adopt or not to adopt the sick role. Their choice is dependent on their social and cultural conditioning as well as their individual ability to cope with the possibility of impending change in their way of life and how they face the possibility of death. Some people may choose to accept the diagnosis of a disease as a death sentence whilst others may view diagnosis as an opportunity to make the most of the remainder of their life. For example; Respondent 9 (COGIC) viewed her breast cancer as an opportunity to prove God and that by sharing her experiences of how she has been healed, the treatment given by the doctors and nurses will help others overcome their fear of breast cancer as a killer disease.

Respondent 9: *It was in 1996 when I was taking a bath and found a lump in my right breast. I went to the doctor who sent me to the hospital they said I would have to have an operation. I had the operation and they said I needed to have more treatment. So I went for the radiotherapy.*
Some years later there I went for a mammogram and there was a shadow on my left breast. They took the lump away and said it was cancerous. They put a drain in and when the drain was taken out there was a lot of fluid in my breast. So I had to go back to my doctor for him to put another drain to remove the excess fluid.
The church prayed. Whilst I was in hospital they visited and prayed. I thank God because if He was not with me and healed me I would not be here today.
When we are not in Church the church pray for us and I believe that through the prayer of the believers God provides healing.
I want to tell others about my experience so that they can have some hope if they are going through similar experiences.

This respondent does not relate her experience of illness and healing directly in the context of suffering. As a result of her belief in the power of prayer she refused to take the sick role that allowed her to stay in hospital or at home. She was excused from her daily activities during her stay in hospital but like most people adopting the sick role and staying in hospital was an acceptable option. Her suffering of pain and discomfort was as short lived as possible. She was eager to get back to church and talk about her healing. On the other hand she may have expected to die as a result of being diagnosed with cancer. Therefore her suffering may have been more intense than if she had immediately accepted that breast cancer is a treatable condition.

According to Wainwright and Calnan (2002) 'signing off sick' has enabled people to opt out of their social responsibilities and in recent years there has been a drive by the Department of Health and the Department of Employment to encourage people who have been on long term sickness benefit to return to work by offering financial incentives. Older people from developing countries such as the Caribbean are not used to the luxury of being paid for being sick. In addition to this, it is regarded as a dishonest action by many church attendees. An added aspect is that the majority of the people will seek spiritual healing so that they can continue to work.

Seeking spiritual healing before going to the doctor for a medical diagnosis means that the person has made his own diagnosis. He has probably chosen not to engage with the illness behaviour suggested in the sick role model. Zola's (1973) typology of the timing of decisions to seek medical intervention showed that many people tolerated symptoms before seeking a diagnosis and treatment from a healthcare professional. Those who perceive themselves to be suffering may respond to external and internal triggers by setting a deadline to feel better. For example they may say "If I don't feel better after church on Sunday I will go to the doctor on Monday". Sunday, being the day when they actively seek prayer or they are rested. What is interesting is that the spiritual healer will advise the person to seek confirmation from their doctor that the condition exists and that the person is not asking for healing for something that is only in their mind. The spiritual healer does not claim to have medical knowledge or to have any knowledge outside of the person seeking healing or their medical practitioner. Once they have attended the doctor and have a diagnosis they then engage with the illness behaviour model. In this situation, as the spiritual healer encourages the input of the medical doctor it is impossible for him to claim alternative therapy for the healing process. He can however claim to be delivering a therapy that is complementary to medicine.

To engage in the act of asking for healing means that the person is accepting the sick role or not accepting the sick role. If the action is before having a medical diagnosis this could be regarded as not adopting the contemporary sick role that Parsons (1975) describes taking action such as seeking prayer or going to the doctor and taking the medicine that is prescribed by the doctor to get better can be either accepting the suffering or not accepting the suffering and enduring (tolerate) pain and illness.

Suffering or the experiences of pain, sorrow, defeat or change cannot be explored without exploring the sick role, health and healing also in a cultural context (c.f Rose 1999). In some cultures mental illness is not acknowledged, probably because the concept of mental illness as a spiritual psychological aspect of the person is regarded as beyond human understanding. These aspects of the person are placed clearly in the domain of the supernatural where an understanding of God and the spirits can possibly explain these phenomena.

Suffering and spirituality in the Caribbean migrant meet in the experiences of isolation through change as they encountered the British people when they first arrived in this country. For some of these Christians, the scars run deep and they vowed not to set foot in the 'white man's church.' Some church attendees will deliberately seek to attend a black majority church, where they feel immediately accepted on the basis of their colour. They are not subjected to the indignity of being told, or being made to feel, that they are in the wrong place. Many elderly members of the Black majority churches do not feel that they have the privilege of attending a white majority church. Consequently they overcome any discomfort that accompanies the changes such as a change of minister or a different approach to the practice of the church doctrine in their church. In addition to this, they request healing from physical conditions but not from psychological conditions. The psychological condition being that of the anger, hurt rejection that they experience. This experience may have reinforced the legacy of slavery when their ancestors were forced out of their environment first, by being taken from their own country and then being sold as chattels (c.f. Austin-Broos 1992). The importation of labour has similar connotations of slavery except that there were promises that their life would be better if they emigrated, as they could work and improve the lives of their family in their birth country. These promises were short lived as the new arrivals met with a hostility that they were not prepared for (Rose 1999).

This hostility brought back memories of the experiences of their forefathers who were bought into slavery. Suffering the pain of hostility and rejection which included being rejected by the white majority churches resulted in seeking to develop their Christianity where they were comfortable within their own community. There were similarities of rejection in schools and the transfer to the labour market.

'Whatever the educational attainment of the black school leaver, he was denied the opportunity to a white collar job.' (Hiro 1991:53) Blauner (1990) shows that the situation was not so different in the United States, where during the 60s black people as a group remained in the lower level earning bracket. Although they were on a high level of employment, they were in a low level for salary. As a consequence of this oppression, the black majority churches also have a high population of low paid workers who subsidise the church from their low pay. The migrants did not intentionally seek to break the inter-generational curse, (cf Hickey 2000) of the legacy of slavery which led them to shun the white person at all costs. They separated work from the rest of their lives and went to work even when they were ill. They were reluctant to take time off work for a mental health problem such as depression as they did not regard this as an illness. Some people adamantly refuse to consult with a white doctor and others will pay for medical care because they believe that by paying they get better and culturally sensitive treatment. They are not accustomed to getting medical care that they do not have pay for. Their suffering is culturally conditioned although for some there may appear similarities with the story of Job. Throughout his suffering, Job did not reject God and maintained his faith in a God that allows suffering for a purpose for those who accepts His will and for those who do not accept His will.

Many church goers in the Black Pentecostal churches like COGIC regard themselves as having suffered through the generations, and especially during their early days in this country. They often testify to the suffering in different forms. The refusal of jobs and housing, and medical care that is not designed for them may compound their suffering and force them to seek spiritual healing. The stresses of unemployment, isolation in the workplace and difficulties in gaining promotion in employment seemed like a contributory factor in the high incidence of hypertension and stroke (Balarajan et al.1989) in Black and ethnic minority populations, a correlation confirmed by the 1991 Census (Raleigh and Balarajan, 1994). Their regular attendance at church, seeking healing through forgiveness as well as physical healing, is indicative of a resilience that vaguely matches the experience of Job. In addition to this there is the issue of suffering as a result of being in a cold country where the climate is as cold as the host population.

During the winter months the average attendance at church services are usually below 50% of the total membership on the grounds of coughs and colds which as Calley (1965), remarked more than forty years ago, may be is sufficient grounds to keep the person at home or in bed. My research shows that there are usually more requests for prayer for sick members and relatives during the winter months. This research also found that the requests for prayer during the winter months were similarly frequent in the URC and COGIC. It may be that things have changed in the forty-five years since Calley's research and there is more parity between the two races and cultures and the churches. Alternatively it may be that there are more young people in the COGIC and more elderly people in the URC. One might speculate that as the incidence of hypertension and stroke is lower for the White British population, it is possible that the level of stress is lower and therefore church attendees do not seek spiritual healing so often for these conditions. They may however, seek spiritual healing or adopt the sick role for other conditions such as cancers.

Drawing on Job as an Example of Suffering

The use of Job as an exemplar of suffering by respondents is parallel in view in its treatment in popular theology. Atkinson (1991) offers a pastoral exploration of Job's story. 'The message of Job is a comfort to us in our own suffering and healing and a model for ministry to others in pain' and Lewis (2003) wrote 'God whispers in our pleasures but shouts in our pain. It is His megaphone that arouses a deaf world.' The author of the book of Job attempts to illustrate the concept of suffering, through an exploration of good and evil and how human beings can and should respond to suffering.

The book of Job presents an imaginative example of suffering and healing which many Christians view as real. The author of Job (Ch.1, vs 6-11) presents God like a King who has a council that includes an impudent being called Satan (an embodiment of cynicism) who doubts that anyone could be God-fearing unless it was in their favour. This scenario by the author enables him to show a healthy mind in a variety of awful situations. When that mind's belief is challenged by the premature death of family, trust in God conflicts with the drive to preserve life at all cost. This drive to preserve life may increase suffering, albeit temporarily. For example, radiation or chemotherapy treatments for cancer often temporarily increase suffering. The drive to preserve or to prolong life may in some situations be more to relieve the suffering of relatives and friends than of the person who is dying. Family and friends are often unable to articulate their inherent need to keep the person alive and express their own needs through the possible needs of the suffering person. Job's wife is a possible example. (Job 2). She was unable to see or to experience what Job was experiencing or to visualize the real outcome of his death, yet she was ready to encourage him to seek death by rejecting God. Job responded by regarding her as speaking *like* a foolish woman which is not the same as saying she is foolish or wrong. Job declares that she is presenting him with a similar option to the situation that he is already experiencing. He does not know what the next day will be like, anymore than he knows what death will be like for him or for her. It could be interpreted that Job's wife was probably a reflection of Job and her words the ones that Job was saying to himself.

Respondent 4's view is that her sister is not suffering because she repeatedly brings misfortune on herself and uses this as excuse to adopt the sick role. Her views have similarities to those of Job's friends who believe that there must be something in Job's life that is not right, therefore he has brought this suffering on himself. Her sister's suffering is not one of innocence in the same way that innocent children die and their parents suffer through their grief as with Job's innocent suffering.

Interviewer: *Do you think some of that is suffering?*

Respondent 4*: Not for my sister she has always managed to get everyone doing things for her throughout her life. She has never actually done very much for herself or anyone else.* (see 6.3 perceptions on suffering)

The Jerome Bible commentators (MacKenzie, and Murphy, 1996) propose that there is nothing in Job's conduct which indicates that his suffering is just, or a punishment for sin. The extent of Job's suffering is so un-believable that although his imaginary friends sat with him in silence, they were not convinced that his suffering was not a result of sin. Eliphaz advised "If you repent Job, then all this will go away and God's blessing will return," Job was not prepared to take the advice because when he searched his own heart he had no guilt and responds 'I would still have this consolation—my joy in unrelenting pain, that I have not denied the words of the Holy One.' The next two friends are of the same opinion that Job was not as righteous as he should be and this is why he was suffering as a punishment. Job remains equally unconvinced and responded in humility by repeating that he has questioned God's purposes and came close to charging God with injustice. His repentance brought him his healing.

The concept of suffering is further developed in the New Testament, as in John 9 where the Pharisees question the cause for the blind man's suffering. Jesus responded that that sin, suffering and healing is addressed by God to His glory. There is a parallel between Job and Christ in that Job suffered and was healed through his humility. Jesus also suffered and gave healing through His humility.

The comments of respondent 10 below quoted in section 6.3 above, "*This period of time allowed me to humble myself . . . .*" also illustrate humility as a contributing factor her healing and relief from her suffering.

Suffering and the Casting out of Spirits

A more radical spiritual interpretation of suffering, or of some suffering, casts it as a direct result of spiritual forces. The interpretations of the book of Job see the heavenly personages as embodiments of human arguments; but they also appear in the discourse of respondents as independent agents. According to James (2001) there is confusion between the medical view (where demonic possession is regarded as hysteria or possible mental illness) and the religious view (where the demonic spirit is interpreted as evil). Although the medical view tries to disentangle itself from religious superstition, they often become entangled and confused on the very point they are trying to clarify. Bourguignon (1976:113) suggests that spirit possession should not be seen as merely a form of cultural theatre, which is different in each society. Nor should spirit possession be seen as just as a form of mental illness, which is the view that scientific medicine has developed toward the phenomenon. She argued that "the neuro-physiological approach could lead to a better understanding of cognition cross-culturally and a method of organizing different phenomena in disparate societies under a common label".

The Christian tradition in both COGIC and (more tenuously) the URC accepts that demonic spirits can manifest themselves in the form of mental illnesses and require healing mediated by an appropriate person. Such spirits are often seen as fallen angels. Demons as well as angels can ascend the heights of spirituality as well as reach the depths of hatred, bitterness and perversion. Prayer can be used to restrain demonic activity as demonstrated in Mark 5 where Jesus ordered the unclean spirits to leave the man in the graveyard. As recorded in verse 12, all the demons begged Him saying 'Send us to the swine that we may enter them.' and the swine ran into the sea and drowned. Demonic spirits in the discourse of some respondents appear as the cause of discomfort or *dis-ease* in the body which has no apparent physical explanation yet cause the person to suffer at varying degree. Christians who are following the example of Christ as outlined in the gospel, are deemed to have unlimited authority over demons and have the authority to exorcise or to command the demon to leave the individual, a house or wherever the demon happens to be.

Such is the mysterious effect of the presence and healing of demons that being mentally unbalanced is taboo in many societies including the West Indian communities and their churches. If a person is emotionally or mentally unbalanced, this is often explained as witchcraft, obeah, black magic or demon possession. It is accepted by the community that prayer can be used to drive out the demons and effect healing. For those who do not attend church on a regular basis, a request may be sent to the church leaders by a family member asking for prayer for the person or the church leader may be asked to visit the person and pray for them. In the words of several respondents who do not view depression as an illness but recognized that there is an imbalance (depression) which could be regarded as demonic or cultural. There was no immediate 'casting out of demonic spirits' but medical treatment of mental imbalance gave the person a sense of balance.

Respondent 11 from COGIC noted:

'I went to the doctor because I could not sleep and my hair was falling out. My husband told me to go and see the doctor because something is wrong. The doctor told me I was depressed because of the diagnosis that my child was severely autistic and gave me some pills' It took two years before I began to feel better.
'Depression does not happen to black folks, only white folks'.

Kaufman, (1996) suggests that when our dignity pride and self worth are undermined, the causes are often attributed to an unacceptable force that is outside of the control of the person. At the same time, that person is expected to be able to regain a balance with or without help, and with the assistance of strong willpower. The person who suffers an unbalanced state for any period of time is labelled a 'lunatic' or 'possessed with demons' and shunned by their family and the community.

Amongst COGIC church members, when one comes to Christ, he or she is healed of any mental or emotional frailty which can be regarded as demonic spirits. When they are healed they leave this aspect of their past lives and these demons behind. They are now renewed to wholeness through the healing power of Christ. They are healed of any past sinful activities such as cussing, stealing, lying and adultery, alcoholism and smoking. Those living with a partner without the sanctity of marriage are expected to marry their partner as a sign of moving to a new and renewed life in Christ. The family is a strong influence in the person's life. Although written policy is not explicit, if the family becomes an obstacle to the person becoming a born again Christian, the family may be abandoned and the person becomes adopted by a church family.

The rule in COGIC is total abstinence from alcohol. Someone who abuses alcohol on a regular basis will not be offered membership status and if they are a member and resort to a 'drunken way of life' they will be excommunicated as this is regarded as a sin and one which is not accepted by the church community, whereas in the URC someone who overuses alcohol and smokes can remain in membership, even as an elder although every effort will be made to help this person overcome their 'demonic' habit.

Mental imbalance as a form of suffering appears to be more accepted in the URC and the presence of mental illness is not a deterrent to membership providing it is not disruptive to the church and it members. Any disruptive behaviour is monitored closely and the person will be asked to refrain from these behaviours. If they do not respond to the request to they will be asked not to attend the services. There is no talk of possession by demonic spirits. The person with a mental imbalance will be referred to a doctor for depression, Alcoholics Anonymous for alcohol abuse or a drug rehabilitation program for drug abuse.

In many human societies, some people believe in spirit possession and this belief can be a fundamental part of the health beliefs. Indeed, if we see poor sanitation, microbes, viruses as possible manifestations of evil and demonic forces; liberal Christians could also argue that suffering, sicknesses and death in Third World countries have been visited on them by demonic forces. Explanations of spirit possession appeared frequently in various historical periods and across many different cultures (Tantam1993; Castillo1997; James 2002). The respondents in this study link it to biblical stories such as in Mark chapter 5 (Vs 1-20).

The extract below from the data illustrates a claim of demonic spirit possession during a service which was suspended for about thirty minutes (unplanned) whilst the demonic spirit was recognized and ministers engaged in a long process of prayer to restore the person to normality.

Observation in a COGIC church service

This lady was sitting in the row of seats behind me.
The previous day she had gone forward for prayer. At the end of the prayer those who had requested prayer were asked for a show of hands if they have decided to accept Jesus as their personal Saviour. This is the first step towards

becoming a member of the Pentecostal church. She testified that there were some obstacles in her life which prevented her from surrendering her life to God. During the service, the majority of the congregation were in an altered state of consciousness and so was this lady. Two ladies who were introduced as ministers earlier in the service were praying with her. The lady fell to the floor and appeared to be in a state of collapse. She was not saying anything. The chanting of 'Praise the Lord,' speaking in tongues and the ritualistic praying over her continued for about twenty minutes whilst the rest of the congregation, including the moderator watched.

As she lay prostrated on the floor there were three ladies praying for her. Her eyes were rolling and she was visibly salivating from the corners of her mouth. She appeared totally oblivious to what was happening in her surroundings. At one point there was some concern as to whether she was breathing as her limbs were floppy and she was not moving. One of the praying ladies asked everyone else to move away from her (to avoid crowding her and to allow those praying some space). Then one lady said 'she is possessed by demons.' During this time the rest of the congregation (about 150 people) looked on and the moderator stopped the service. After about twenty minutes of animated activities by the praying ladies around the prostrate lady, the prostrate lady appeared more conscious and was assisted from the service by the praying ladies who continued to pray for her in an adjoining room. The moderator then continued the service.

About thirty minutes later the praying party and the 'spirit possessed' lady rejoined the service. This she did as though nothing unusual had happened as she was not aware that the service was stopped for thirty minutes because the spirit was dealing with her. The lady later testified that she has been released from the obstacles which had prevented her from surrendering her life to God. Throughout the encounter, the person looked uncomfortable as though she was really suffering.

It was not possible to ascertain if there was indeed spirit possession and there was no indication outside the prayer session that such was the case with this lady. It did appear that she was experiencing an internal conflict and this could be reminiscent of Jung's (1959) speculations about demon possession. Jung (1959: 323-324) postulated that possessing spirits directly relates to archetypes. "It may even happen that the archetypal figures, which are endowed with a certain autonomy anyway on account of their luminosity, will escape from conscious control altogether and become completely independent, thus producing the phenomenon of possession".

In the observation example quoted above it was not the Pastor who was praying for the 'demon possessed' person. It was not the moderator who recognized the needs of this person; it was members of the congregation who believed that they had the power and the authority to pray with her. Influencing them may have been the readily available work of the evangelist Munroe (2002) who asserts that "We must be able to legally use the authority behind the power of Jesus to obtain results in prayer" citing the violent confrontation that Peter had with the evil or demonic spirit in Acts 19. The Pastor and the moderator accepted the power and authority of these praying women and allowed the service to be interrupted so that this person could receive prayer for healing.

As noted above, Bourguignon (1976: 113) warns that we should not fail to look for common neuro-physiological processes in cases of spirit possession, whatever our own view of their cultural construction. The spirit which possessed the person in Mark 5 appeared to be self-destructive as he was in the mountains "cutting himself with stones" and ran to worship Jesus as well as denouncing Him. This suggests the possibility of an abnormal mental state, a personality disorder or, in psychological terms, a psychotic illness. In spiritual terms it is possible that there was a disturbed spirit where healing and wholeness can be afforded to the sufferer through the intervention of Jesus.

Healing from the Suffering of Rejection

We have discussed above how psychological rejection causes an emotional imbalance and therefore a homeostatic physical imbalance in varying degrees. The emotional response to pain is subjective and cannot be easily explained. The causes of suffering may be hidden, as in the multiple legacies of slavery addressed above, which may give rise to the notion of a special 'Black pathology' (c.f. Toulis 1997). In addition to this, adults who have experienced abuse as children may live with its memory suppressed and without a deep subconscious healing and a conscious effort to engage in forgiveness of the perpetrators.

Health Promotion—Spiritual Healing

Respondent 11 (COGIC) indicated that suffering took the form of a void in her life, which could almost be called an open wound. Her mother had died when she was born. She experienced a deep sense of rejection before she was made conscious that her mother died at her birth.

Her story: *'My father died before I was born and my mother died the day I was born. I did not know that the woman who raised me was not my mother till I was in my thirties. During a healing session I went for prayer for healing. During the prayer I was told to forgive my mother. This was puzzling to me as I was not holding anything against mother. I appreciate all that my adopted mother had done for me and accepted the explanation that was given to me about my biological mother. Another person offered to represent my mother and apologized for not being there for me. She said 'I am sorry for not being there to feed you, provide shelter and clothing for you, for not being there to take you to school and for all the other things a mother would do for her child' During the session I was extremely tearful but after the experience I felt that a weight had been lifted from me. I felt that the missing link of my life was replaced.*

The interpretation, which had been arrived at, was that the child continued to be connected to the mother spiritually and emotionally and suffered the loss of her mother although she did not realize this on a conscious level. It addresses speculations about whether the person who raised the child had a different method of child rearing to that which would have been employed by the mother had she lived. Very importantly it addressed the consequences of the child not having been told that her mother had died when she was born and that someone else has provided everything for her (shelter, food, clothes education, and love) and so there was still something missing in her life.

There is some indication that during the experience of the healing process someone identified the void and replaced this with an apology and a physical presentation of her biological mother (by pretending to be her biological mother). This interaction took her back to the consciousness of her birth, possibly imaginary and also said words of apology that she wanted to hear and she understood.

The physical representation of the situation provided a reality for the void that she now felt had existed throughout her life and helped her to identify what was missing from her life and the reason for her suffering. Thus she began to experience the healing process. She was healed from rejection through a process that is similar to the way that healing from a physical wound occurs, as illustrated in detail in the literature review chapter. The tears could be compared to the flow of pus and lymph fluids, which is also a cleansing process.

Although she was not consciously aware of the separation from her mother till late in her life, the physical acknowledgement of her emotional pain and the verbal recognition of the missing elements in her life enabled her to acknowledge the pain and allowed her to be relieved of the burden and suffering of rejection.

She was thus consciously able to forgive her mother for 'rejecting and abandoning' her as a baby. Seeking forgiveness is a way to relieve suffering. Lucas (1997), in the introduction to his collection, postulates that in seeking forgiveness the sufferer may have been wronged in reality or perception and this may add to the pain of the illness. Lucas believes that we are instructed to forgive one another partly to release the offender but also for healing of the offended. In the URC, the minister enables members of the congregation to seek this level of forgiveness by directly inviting them to ask individually and collectively for forgiveness, in the spirit of Jesus who was unjustly tried, suffered and put to death, yet before he died he said 'Father forgive them for they do not know what they are doing' (Luke 23).

It is sometimes difficult to overcome bitterness, guilt and to forgive oneself for causing suffering to another person and even more difficult to forgive others for causing suffering to oneself. Planting the seed of forgiveness starts with blessing the person to be forgiven, and therefore gives space for the process of grace and faith in the power of forgiveness to start working on oneself. Through suffering, the Christian church demonstrates the power of the powerless to the world in the face of its oppressors. Christian faith is not just a proclamation of faith; it is active moral striving in a hostile world.

The healing effect of positive emotions may have the potential to reduce stress on the cardiovascular system (Banner 2001, Witvleit et al. 2001). In contrast, a pattern of infrequent negative emotional arousal or one that rapidly return to a calm baseline following negative arousal could have a beneficial effect on health.

It may therefore be true to say that prayer produces positive emotions, a positive approach to any situation reduces stress on the cardiovascular system, allows the body space to deal with physical internal stress thus relieving suffering and contribute to the process of healing. Worthington et al. (2007) posit that positive responses are essential aspects of emotional experiences, countering emotional responses such as grudges. People may feel wretched and guilty in holding a grudge towards another person who mistreated, offended or hurt them. Witvleit et al (2001) suggest that reduction in hostility brought about by behavioural intervention that encourages forgiveness can reduce coronary problems. Where people hold a grudge, they stay in the victim role and perpetuate negative emotions associated with the hurtful offence and the experience of suffering. Contributors to Tugwell et al (1976) postulate that spiritual healing can come through the deep fellowship found in the type of worship similar to that of the Azuza Street revival, especially when, contrary to the previous American (or British) norm, it was interracial. As suggested in Chapters Four and Five above, this type of worship enables the person to move away from the negative emotions and hurtful experience of suffering as experienced by black people as a legacy of slavery.

Death can be regarded as a state of rejection and ultimate suffering or healing for the person who has died and for their relatives. As ultimate healing, this can be a welcomed relief from the suffering of an illness such as rheumatoid arthritis, cancers and diseases that cause breathing difficulties. The professional and personal experiences of the researcher as a counsellor and a believer in Christian healing indicate that people who have a belief in God and His healing powers experience suffering with a certain level of joy. Those who experience the separation that accompanies death cope better than those without an active faith and belief in healing. Those without a faith and belief in a supernatural being are more emotionally traumatized and at a higher risk of having reactive mental health problems as described in Holmes-Rahe social adjustment scale (Holmes and Rahe 1967).

Grieving is a psychological process wherein emotional wounds are either healed or fail to be healed. The process is similar to the healing of a physical wound. Some physical wounds heal spontaneously without medical intervention or wound care. Larger and deeper wounds need medical intervention to aid the healing process and take a longer time to heal. In the same way larger psychological trauma require a longer grieving time. Sometimes sufferers can be assisted or accelerated by counselling support, prayer and social support from relatives and friends. Social support from relatives and friends can be supplemented by the church family or as a family-friendly environment like the one at the Wellbridge centre for the elderly. At the Wellbridge resource centre, the elderly clients who have experienced many psychological traumas highlighted how the centre helped them to lead happy and relaxed lives The centre provides residential care, day care, outreach home care physiotherapy, occupational therapy, and speech, music and dance therapy which aid the healing process (Jeffries 2003).

Anger, bitterness and hatred could paralyze them emotionally and spiritually, prevent their progress and engage with the hurt, pain and suffering. By using therapeutic touch, prayer and the laying of hands enable the person to claim deep healing as the healing by secondary intention. This could be through a slow process or quickly as by a 'miracle'. The decision as to whether this is a slow process or a quick 'miracle' in Pearce's (2005) sense, depends on the lesson that persons have to learn and how well they learn this lesson. Recurrence of a wound that has been healed through prayer can take place in the same way that a physical wound breaks down when healing was superficial initially. Superficial healing of a physical wound takes place when scar tissue forms over the wound but the deeper section of the wound is not healed. Suffering from one of the deeper psychological wounds comes through the experience of loss, bereavement and grief as will be illustrated in the account of a young mother in the next section.

Breaking the Generational Cycle of Suffering

Hickey (2000) suggests that if a person grows up in a home where parents were emotionally unhealthy it is more likely that the child will fall in the same emotional traps when they become parents. The possible outcomes of unhealthy emotions are alienation severe depression and nervous breakdown; and the beginning of healing of unhealthy emotions is forgiveness. In my observation notes there is the following example:.

A young mother in (URC) told the researcher her story of how she had been sexually assaulted by her father for many years. There was an investigation, but he was not prosecuted because there was not enough evidence. The father did not believe that he had done anything wrong.

She now has two children of her own and is expecting a third child. The father of her children recently left her and the family home for another woman. Her father had no access to her children (his grand children). She said 'I will not allow my father to see my children unsupervised.' Although this caused her some concern she had resigned herself that this was for the best, but if the children wanted to see their grandfather when they were old enough to look after themselves she would not object. She felt that she had a responsibility to teach the children that if someone touched them inappropriately they would have the courage to tell her or another adult. She was adamant that she did not want her children to go through the same experience as she and her twin sister. Both girls had been told categorically by their father that this was their secret and consequently they did not think that this was wrong until they went to school and realized that their friends did not have the same experiences and that this parental behaviour was inappropriate. She admitted that she was going through a difficult time and she would like some help.

As she related her story, her suffering seemed so intense that as a mother I wanted to hold her, be there for her, and provide some comfort (healing) for her. My own thoughts about healing at this time were influenced by the popular pastoral theology of Hickey (2000) about breaking the cycle of abuse through the 'Breaking the generational curse'. Hickey wrote: 'Doctors are aware that physical afflictions can be the result of a generational iniquity. When you show signs of certain types of diseases, they want to know if there is a family history of that disease. Maybe arthritis, diabetes, or heart disease runs in your family.' Hickey postulates that down the generations, "curse sickness" may be caused by someone doing another person an injustice or wickedness and that injustice may be visited on the children from the parents through generations. She cites

Psalms 103:3 'who forgiveth all thine inequities: who healeth thy diseases' and Isaiah 'and the inhabitants shall not say I am sick; the people that dwell therein shall be forgiven for their iniquity' and 'He was wounded for our trespasses and bruised for our iniquities'. In these scriptures, sickness/healing is linked with iniquity.

What is interesting about this young mother's story is that her father did not believe that what he did was wrong because his father had also abused him. The type of healing that this young mother required was one of first and second intention or deep centred healing. The young mother had started to take steps towards breaking the generational cycle, but she was still suffering. Her children would suffer in a lesser form from this particular curse by not having a normal relationship with their grandfather during their developing years. Eventually she had taken steps to heal the rift by allowing the children to see their grandfather under supervision. This required a deep centred healing, one that in my view would be miraculous and probably not easily explainable. She required a strategy and a feasible explanation for using this strategy of supervised access. However she has taken certain actions to keep her children safe and to break the 'generation curse'. The experience of forgiveness for her father does not appear to have taken place with this young mother although the process of breaking the generation curse has begun. It may be that even when this young mother has forgiven her father, the breaking of the generational curse will involve a change in the emotional relationship with the mother and her father so that she can protect her own children.

Hickey (2000) goes on to say that the blood of Jesus is all sufficient, powerful and devastating to family iniquities in your heritage. Positive thinking like counselling, even doing religious things like singing in the choir, whilst good, will not solve the problem. They may provide temporary relief, but only the blood of Jesus is the permanent answer, transforming your curse into a blessing. The comments and experiences of respondent 11 illustrates some similarities with Hickey's views on suffering and healing, that Jesus has the power to heal.

The view of forgiveness held by Witvleit et al (2001) provides a psychological exposition of the effects of forgiveness on the physical and psychological body comparing religious and humanist perspectives. They suggest the humanists' emotional experience of non—forgiveness and forgiveness are very similar to the Christian experiences, in line with the teaching of Christ and the apostles.

For this young mother the process of forgiveness has begun. She had also made some progress in the process of forgiveness and the breaking of the generation curse by stating that 'I will not allow my father to see my children unsupervised. She did not say 'I will not allow my father to see my children (his grand children).' She recognized the importance of allowing her children access to their grandfather and at the same time allowing him to understand that she will not allow them to have similar experiences to hers, when she was abused by him. There is some evidence that she has started to forgive her father as she expressed a wish for her father to have supervised access to his grandchildren.

Conclusion

Perceptions of suffering, physical and psychological pain are culture bound, yet within the context of culture there are individual interpretations. This is futher highlighted by Parsons' sick role model and possibly the availability of economic and religious (spiritual) interpretations for sickness, illness and disease. Consequently spiritual healing from the pains of suffering is also culturally and economically sanctioned. Suffering may be attributed to generational 'curse' or 'cure' where the person or their family make a concerted effort to move away from'the curse' of an illness is due to a particular condition such as alcoholism in the family or to accept that this will not continue to the next generation. Perception of suffering is inextricably interwoven with faith and is also closely linked to the doctrine of both churches. Both churches use translations of the Nicene creed as the foundation for their faith and their belief in spiritual healing. Although perception of suffering is culturally bound as well as individualistic, it is a common human experience and not related to any one cultural, religious experience which is expressed at different levels.

Suffering and its complex relationship to faith is often wrestled with in the health promotion activities of prayer, laying of hands and music used to aid spiritual healing in both churches. These activities are discussed in more details in Chapters 4, 5, and 6.

Chapter Four

Prayer as a Healing Activity

Introduction

This chapter explores the ethnographic findings on how prayer is regularly used in the delivery of spiritual healing in the two churches and to interrogate and attribute meaning to this evidence. It also presents extracts from interviews under the headings of how the churches pray for healing, prayer for specific illnesses, distant healing versus contact healing and discusses how prayer links with models of health as presented in the sociology of health and used in the NHS by professionals health care workers. This leads to a discussion on how prayer is used in spiritual healing and the perceived outcomes for those who deliver and receive prayer. Dossey (1997), Byrd (1998) and Narayansamy and Narayansamy (2008), outline, illustrate and contextualise the social processes on how prayer can be seen as an independent variable affecting health outcomes.

Prayer is used in both churches under study as a health seeking behaviour as well as a worship activity. In the URC, prayer for healing is focused during prayers of intercession and there is also a special service where the whole service if focused on healing, which concludes with prayer and the 'laying on of hands' by the minister and elders for anyone who wishes to take this opportunity to receive a focused prayer. Seeking prayer is not given as one of the examples of health seeking behaviour which constitutes conformity to the sick role in Parsons' (1975) original discussion. Nonetheless when a the person seeking prayer steps out in a public way to say 'I am not well and therefore I am seeking prayer to make me better', as though prayer were a therapy, we can look at the factors leading to this behaviour within models derived from the more empirical studies of social responses by the individual to illness from Dingwall (1976) to Weiss and Lonnquist (2005).

The findings show how prayer is used in distant healing and contact healing in the two churches in the study. There are differences, however. In the Pentecostal church prayer for healing is not separated from prayer for repentance, sanctification, justification and becoming a born again Christian. It is always present because, since Pentecostal eschatology suggests we are already living in "the end times", and so Christians can always claim the possibilities of healing right now. For the URC, while Christians may always ask for healing, they accept it may not arrive until we are all in heaven, so healing services are something extra to normal everyday Christian worship in this world. There is no evidence that the differences in the services have different outcomes, although Dossey (1997) maintains that an impressive body of evidence suggests that prayer and religious devotion are associated with positive health outcomes.

Unsurprisingly, there are also gender and ethnicity-related variations. Levin and Schiller (1987) found that generally in the USA females and African Americans prayed more frequently than those who are males and white. The majority of church attendees in both URC and COGIC in my study happen to be female and black. There is also a similarity in those who volunteered to be interviewed. However, these results may be related to the geographical location where the study was conducted and cannot be generalised even in other areas where black and ethnic minority population represent the majority ethnic group.

Purpose of Prayer

Prayer is at the heart of Christian life and is seen as a two way communication that creates a conscious relationship with God, in whatever way God is understood. Rice and Huffstattler (2001) assert that it is not a mindless task and places demands on those who pray. These demands include an expectation of an outcome, to be genuine in supplication. There is a requirement for subjective sincerity and honesty in prayer, although honesty is sometimes painful. The private prayers of individuals prepare them for public prayers. Rahner (1982) reminds us that each day millions of people take time to pray; some take hours and some may take only a few minutes.

The leadership of both congregations see prayer as contributing to providing a psychological environment that could be regarded as therapeutic and safe, one that can restore harmony and also contribute to the healing process. Hospitals and doctors' surgeries can be regarded as places of quarantine from normal social support networks and therefore places of stress, although prayer can contribute to making them a healing environment. Those taking part in spiritual healing tend, by contrast, to see religious buildings where spiritual activities are performed, as therapeutic, safe and healing environments. In using the medium of prayer, spiritual healing can be administered as distant or contact healing as illustrated in the two churches.

Non-academic, or 'popular' Christian writers such as Munroe (2001:36-37), suggest prayer 'is the expression of man's relationship with God and participation in his purposes', patterned on the Garden of Eden when God made a practice of walking and talking with Adam. (Genesis 3). The theologian Stacey (1977) argues that a new kind of prayer brought Jews and Gentiles together in worship in the corporate life of the early church, and was reckoned to be the privilege of those who had put on Christ and received the Spirit. Prayer is also defined and explored as a declaration of faith as well as to reinforce a personal relationship with a divine or superior being.

Some form of prayer is articulated in most religions and cultures which postulate a supernatural deity or deities, although prayer still remains a mysterious activity. to the believer, the atheist and the agnostic. Within popular piety, 'prayer is the natural language of religious and cultural experiences' and nursing authors Hawley and Irurita (1998) suggest this is of value in medical practice.

The Christian theologians' typologies of prayer feed through into popular religiosity and influence patterns of prayer, peoples' understandings of how it ought to be done. However natural and spontaneous it may be claimed to be, within these congregations prayer is an activity both learnt, and consciously theorised. Rice and Huffstattler (2001:111-127) describe prayer as having a fourfold nature; adoration confession/pardon, thanksgiving and supplication (or petition). Writing more specifically about the health context in the Journal of Holistic Nursing, Hughes (1997) uses a simpler typology to refer to prayer as supplicative or meditative and infers that prayer presents as communication with a superior being whose capabilities exceed that of human beings and who is willing to give ear to our supplications. The typology of prayer of Rice and Huffstattler is primarily aimed at ministers in the URC. This typology includes the supplicative and meditative prayer referred to by Hughes (1997).

In the URC it is usually the minister who uses the typology verbally to express the needs of the congregation and others, whilst in COGIC any member of the congregation is allowed to say prayer in public with members of the congregation audibly agreeing with the person praying. In the URC the congregation agrees with the minister silently. This approach is also used in healing and services not specific to healing in both churches. Intercessory prayer, according to Robert et al (2009), takes into account the nature of God as all powerful and the nature of man as subjective to the nature of God. In other words, the healer pleads with God as he is subject to God whom he believes to be all powerful. Prayers for healing some else are by definition intercessory and the healer may pray or ask another person to pray (intercede) for him to be used a channel through which the healing power from God can flow. Intercessory prayer is showing compassion for others and can be both meditative and supplicative.

Meditative and supplicative prayer is defined by Hughes (1997) involves a prayer sandwich where in meditative prayer the focus is on the Superior Being, acknowledging Him as the Creator and this is followed by supplicative prayer where the person make a request of the Superior Being and concludes by allowing the Superior Being to respond as he chooses. This is sometimes in the form of giving thanks for answering the prayer in whatever way He chooses. Wagner (1992) espouses the importance of intercessory prayer by and for Pastors and Christian leaders and others such as spiritual healers. He outlines the vulnerability, due to psychological pressures, of spiritual leaders and the need for their own healing so that they can heal others. Wagner (1992) advocates that when the healer petitions God in prayer, it is not only to ask for heavenly things but also to be realistic about their own needs and the needs of others.

Prayer is often used as therapy to replace or to supplement drugs used for physical or psychological (depression) pain. In seeking prayer for healing the person feels that someone is listening to and taking note of their pain.

Depression is not necessarily a mental illness but may be a sane response to the reality of the sufferer's life which is at the time being inappropriately treated by drugs such as prozac, valium or other psychotropic drugs (Lynch 2004). Lynch cites some interesting case histories which show that patients gained far more by having someone listen to them and not judge or blame them, who made them feel safe, recognizing there may be a very good reason why they might feel depressed or suicidal. Seeking prayer and spiritual healing provide a listening ear in a non—judgmental way for those who choose this method. Lynch points to a ray of light and hope in the dark tunnel of mental anxiety in the same way that prayer that is external to the person provides a hope in a situation that the person perceives as hopeless. Other ways of non-chemical mood enhancement include music, as discussed in Chapter 9.

Prayer as Health Seeking Behaviour: How and When the Churches and Individuals Pray for Healing

The idea of prayer for health is widely diffused. "Psychic guru and western Yoga Master" Lawrence (2001) is convinced by the results of a poll conducted for Newsweek 2000, where large majorities of American Catholics, evangelicals, protestants non-Christians and people of no faith say they have prayed to God or a saint for a miracle. In praying for health, members of these congregations are not doing anything particularly unusual. The popular practice, however, overlaps with the theologically defined ritual activity. McCullough (1995) suggests that although the Lord's Prayer encourages them to pray for themselves and others, the primary goal of Christian prayer is to commune with God rather than to improve one's health. The findings of my research show both parameters of communing with God and improving health.

There is a complex relationship between the involvement of faith groups within the NHS, and the practice of private prayer and prayer in church. It is not overtly acknowledged by many doctors of conventional medicine that many patients rely on the prayer of the church to support them through any illness ranging from a minor cold to major surgery or treatment for cancer. Writing about the work of NHS chaplains, however, Kendal-Raynor (2008) argues spiritual assessment should form part of holistic care and prayer should be part of nursing care if the patient's spiritual needs are identified. However, they assert prayer should not be forced on patients and staff should not be forced to pray for patients. This is acknowledged also by popular religious advocates such as Packer and Nystrom (2006), who postulate that the practice of prayer, though a Christian duty, is also a privilege and joy, but not something which can or should be forced. When performed with wisdom and sincerity, they argue that it leads us through different moods and types of praying as well as pointing us to a clearer understanding of the character of God.

Nonetheless, Ewles and Simnett (1999, 2003) and Seedhouse (1997), in their standard health promotion texts, both discuss the spiritual and philosophical aspect of promoting health and the ways in which hospitals and other NHS institutions promote spiritual health in different forms. Some drugs such as those for hormone replacement, pain killers, antibiotics, and psycho-tropic drugs suppress the immune system and can cause depression. Where there is a spiritual aspect to treating these patients and promoting their health, their recovery is likely to be hastened.

The majority of church attenders and spiritual healers in the churches, such as the subjects of the present study, do not exclude conventional medical treatment from prayer as a contribution to health and well being, but treat them as complementary. This is not always the case, however. Peters (2008:112-113) narrates several accounts of when prayer appeared to fail. In one account David's parents Edward and Ann Cornelius took him to a physician who prescribed insulin for his juvenile onset diabetes. He made a good recovery when he adhered to the regular schedule of insulin injections. Although the parents were told that would die without regular schedule of insulin, they refused to heed this advice choosing to treat their son's diabetes by only employing the techniques of their religious faith of praying. This failed, his condition deteriorated and he died. His parents were charged and found guilty of manslaughter and wilful neglect. One of their defences was that medical doctors did not always cure patients and sometimes patients who are undergoing medical intervention die. The suggestion in Peters (2008) that if prayer fails to work it is no different from when medical treatment fails is not sustainable if medical advice has been neglected.

Prayer as a health seeking behaviour, like all health seeking behaviours, includes activities performed in a way that is accepted to the healer and person seeking healing. The passages below explore the effectiveness of the how, when, and where of prayer.

There are three effective classical prayer positions in worship according to Canadian Sufi Muslim mystic 'Raven Rowanchilde' (2003) who outlines them as prostrate face down on the floor, kneeling and standing up. He claims that healing begins when we stand up completely, breathe deeply, raise our hands above our heads and experience the life giving spirit. This resembles to some extent the prayer position of the Pentecostal churches and COGIC.

The position that is usually adopted in the URC, is one of sitting down, crouching the shoulders and bowing the head while the eyes are closed. The older members of the congregation call this the "Congregational crouch" (after the former denominational name, although this "attitude of prayer" differs little from that in other mainstream nonconformist denominations, such as Baptists and Methodists.) The prayer positions in the Pentecostal churches are more varied, from standing with raised hands, standing with heads bowed, kneeling or sitting with head bowed or hands open upwards and raised. However, the prayer position that the respondents or their healers adopted varied in both COGIC and the URC. The positions included kneeling, standing up, walking about, open posture, standing, the congregational crouch, but never a conscious prostrate face down position.

In COGIC, the persons seeking prayer may find themselves on the floor but this was not a deliberate or conscious act. Usually this position is unexplained by the person adopting the position. This position is called 'slain in the spirit' and is more likely to be seen in COGIC than in the URC. Indeed, within the popular religious literature of Pentecostalism there is a critique of positions like the "Congregational crouch" as showing lethargy in praying, failing to encourage the person to receive the energy that is available through a positive act of asking in faith. Selwyn Hughes (2003) in his popular bible-reading notes asserted that many people do not receive from God because they do not ask, and one of these requests should be to help us to pray to overcome lethargy in praying.

From the collected data for this study using the Nvivo coding system Prayer is mentioned 217 times in 24 documents on observations and interviews. From the interviews and the observations, I have selected the contextual use of the term to illustrate the use of prayer in spiritual healing in different interactions and between different individuals.

In the Pentecostal church, prayer for healing is not separated from prayer for repentance, sanctification, justification and becoming a born again Christian. This observation is supported by Paris (1985) and Beckford (2006). In the URC prayer for healing is focused during general congregational prayer that is led by the minister or another person appointed by the minister before the service. There is also a healing service where the whole service is focused on healing and concludes with prayer and the 'laying on of hands' by the minister and elders for anyone who wishes to take this opportunity to have a focused prayer.

Looking at biblical exposition in Christian literature and observations during data collection, prayer appears to be the second most important aspect of spiritual healing.

The most important aspect is the ability of the healer to provide a safe internal and external environment using self and others. In doing so s/he constantly uses the skills of intuition and discernment to channel spiritual energy for the benefit of others. The interaction between the healer and the person seeking healing is a unique and special one which may or may not result in healing. In the churches, the healers pray for guidance, protection, the power and authority of the Holy Spirit, not forgetting the person who is seeking healing. Their prayers sometimes include a request for the approval and authority of the wider church. Prayers are said in different styles of responsive, praying together where the leader initiates the prayer and others participate in groups of men, women or individually. Members of the prayer group or congregation may be asked to describe their concerns as a request for prayer for an individual or a particular situation. Extempore prayers may be made in response to written requests and open prayer allows everyone to make their own contribution.

Harvey (2004) proposes that Jesus' instruction to his disciples on how to pray was a gesture to oppose the Jewish traditional method of praying and a move away from elaborate prayers they were expected to recite every day. In the Lord's Prayer there is an element of petitioning for healing by asking for forgiveness.

Respondent 5 explained her belief in the power of healing that she claimed through her own prayer and fasting.

Respondent 5 (COGIC): *When I received spiritual healing—mmm. When you believe you can. A long time ago, I had a stomach ulcer which lasted years. I went to the hospital, I did everything and I think one day I decided that—and I said 'God if you are really there I am going to fast five days and I want you to heal me.' So I fasted five days without water or food. I just stayed there reading my bible and praying and you know when you have stomach ulcer you have to eat regularly. During the five days I did not have any pain or anything. After the five days I said I was going to eat something that I am not supposed to eat. You know that we Africans, we eat hot peppery and spicy food and you know that plantain can be very hard. So I said I am going to eat hot pepper and roast plantain and that is what I ate. Under normal circumstances when you are fasting, you eat something that is soft, but because I was challenging God, that was what I ate and from there on I have not experienced any pain, I was not rushed to hospital. So I received that healing without going to anybody, just talking to HIM and challenging HIM so I said 'God if you are there I am going to challenge you because you are the healer and I am going to do this through fasting and prayer'.*
I did what an ulcer patient should not do and I got my healing.

Levenstein (1998) gives a bio-medical explanation of gastric or stomach ulcer as understood to be exacerbated by stress as anxiety causes an increase in the production of acidic gastric juices that digest the stomach walls and cause ulcers. During the fasting she rested the stomach and prayer helped her to relax the muscles of the body. Although this is a contradiction to the medical treatment for ulcers it may be that her body had its own way of responding to treatment and one of the reasons for the successful response could be simply allowing the body to rest. What is not easily explained is the permanency of the 'cure'. She did not report a change in her lifestyle, what she did mention was a different approach (possibly cultural) to the usual medical approach for a white European person. Doctors such as Posner (1995) have also explained how this type of response might appear to be a spontaneous remission from a mis-diagnosed cancer.

Respondent 5 account continues where someone prayed for her and where she prayed for another person where she believed healing took place:

When someone prayed for me!!! I have had prayer for minor illnesses such as cold, or headache; I have been anointed with oil and prayed for. I remember once I was coughing, I went to the doctor and the coughing did not stop. I went to church and the minister said we have to anoint you and pray over you so they anointed me and prayed over me. It did not stop immediately. I think it strengthened my faith as I had to go to the doctor again. And when I went to the doctor he prescribed antibiotics and I did not have to take them.
Interviewer: *Have you administered spiritual healing to anyone?*
Respondent: *Oh! A friend of mine came here one day and said uncle was very ill he was rushed to hospital. He had a mild stroke—He was in pain so I said let us go and see him. So we went and he was crawling, he was in so much pain. I did not go with the intention of praying for him but just before we left 'I felt something say 'pray for him', so I asked 'Would you mind if I pray for you?' He said he did not mind. So I just prayed. I laid my hand on him and prayed and he started dancing. It was so instant that I was surprised myself. I don't understand how these things work.*

Asking for healing is demonstrated in the extract in section 6.9 where Respondent 11 explained how she asked for and received healing through her own initiative and in contrast to the doctor's prescription and expectation. Respondent 11 extended her belief in healing for herself to healing for others and was clearly responding to teaching from ministers like Harris (2002)[1]. The laying of hands also allows the person needing

---

[1] Rev Peter Harris (2002) sets out the following five reasons why Christians should pray for healing: Jesus healed the sick; Jesus commanded his disciples

healing to receive the power of the Holy Spirit simultaneously with healing. The above extracts illustrate that faith as well as some confidence in the Christian doctrine, the healer and the power of the Holy Spirit are reasons why Christians pray for themselves, seek the prayer of others and pray for others to be healed. This notion agrees with Harris' views on the reasons why Christians should pray for healing.

The services in COGIC are not specifically focused on healing. Below are two extracts from observation of COGIC services which indicates a similar closing for all the services. An invitation for prayer is made. Those who come forward for prayer is requesting prayer for different things such as healing, the anointing of the Holy Spirit, a deeper understanding of their Christian faith or prayer for another person.
The extract below illustrates the spontaneity of how healing is introduced into COGIC services.

The service began with the usual praise and worship led by the praise and worship team and moderated by one of the younger members (a church elder) Two young people were invited to give an exhortation. This was followed by the collection of the offering (collected in large straw baskets.) During the collection of the offering the praise and worship team sang.
There is a prayer and healing session where the moderator invites the congregation to claim healing by placing their hand on the pain and pray, thus claiming their healing. This continues for about 10 minutes. During this time the majority of the congregation appears to be in state of animation which accompanies an altered state of consciousness as in hysteria
This was followed by a gospel song by the youth choir. The host Pastor greeted the church and then introduced the dignitaries in the congregation to the church. The host minister was also asked to pray for the preacher and introduced the preacher for the day to the congregation.
The preacher greeted the church and introduced the scriptures (2 Samuel 4, 1 Chronicles 16:4 and 2 Chronicles 5:11 matt 21:10.
The topic of the message was workmanship. Throughout the sermon he focused on the young people by consistently making reference to 'young people'

---

to continue His healing ministry The early church healed the sick; Christians through history have healed the sick; The promises of Jesus encourage us.

(1 Samuel 6) he read the whole chapter. A member of the congregation was propelled into shouting and praising God periodically during the delivery of the sermon which lasted 45 minutes

After the sermon (they call this the word or the message for the day) there was an invitation for prayer for healing the baptism of the Holy Spirit, sanctification deliverance from demonic spirits. The invitation is not specific. It is targeted at anyone who needs prayer for whatever the need may be. Several people responded to the invitation and came forward for prayer. All the ministers were invited to pray alone and at the same time for those who came for prayer.

The Pastor invited the church secretary to announce the notices. The Pastor closes the service with a final prayer.

Healing services in the URC are more focused and differentiated from "normal" services.

The sermon continued for about 15-20 minutes

Then there was the call for volunteers to have healing through the laying of hands. The service leader then recalled his experience of a service where he said 'someone in the meeting has a problem from when very young and this is to do with forgiveness. After the service a young man came to him and confessed he had fallen out with his mother at a very young age and had never forgiven her.'

This session took a different approach where the volunteers were asked to show their hands and the ministers would come to them in the congregation and lay hands on them and pray. The congregation was invited to raise their hands, point to the prayer team and the volunteer and pray with them. The musician was asked to play the song 'Be still and know that I am God' from the regularly used hymn book.

Below is an extract from the observation of a URC healing service where the minister conducted the prayer in tongues:

The second minister went forward and they prayed quietly together whilst the congregation looked on and joined quietly in prayer if they so wished.

The organist played quiet background music throughout the healing service. Seven members of the congregation went forward for prayer and laying of hands. Initially two people went forward and each of them was prayed for individually by the ministers both laying hands on each person and prayed.

Dr. Gwen Rose

The first minister prayed in tongues. The other members went forward and each person was prayed for individually.

During the prayers for healing a person may use the gift of tongues to pray as Respondent 2 suggests.

Respondent 2 (URC) said *'If you have the gift of tongues, you can use it during a healing session'. To pray in tongues is to have communication with God that is only understood by the initiated, those who can interpret tongues. This is the time when the healer will be told what to pray for and how to pray although the person seeking prayer and healing may be seeking healing for something else.'*

In a brief interview with a member who attended the prayer meetings and at the end of one meeting this conversation took place. The conversation indicates that there is a belief that the gift of healing is afforded to some people and not to others. In this extract she indicates that Benny Hinn, an international evangelist, has the 'gift'. It is not clear whether she meant the gift of tongues or the gift of healing.

Extract from a conversation with a church member following a COGIC prayer meeting (fieldnote1)

Respondent (not formally interviewed): *What are you studying? Do you visit all the churches?*
Interviewer: *I am looking at the church's approach to spiritual healing. People go to hospital and the church prays for them to be healed. Church members and the minister visit people in hospital and pray for healing for those who are sick. I want to find out how all of this works and what people have to say about it all. It appears that people do not really like to talk about spiritual healing although they pray for the sick.*
Respondent: *You have to have the gift*
Interviewer: *Really!! But the whole church prays for the sick and supports the minister who is praying.*
Respondent: *You have to have faith; People like Benny Hinn pray for people.*

The respondent did not answer the enquiry about spiritual healing and prayer. This was probably because she did not want to expose her lack of knowledge or she did not want to say something that might give a negative view of herself or her church. Instead she attempted to redirect the conversation by the reply "You have to have the gift.''

The researcher tried to get a focus by saying 'the whole church prays for the sick and supports the minister who is praying.' The respondent again redirected the conversation by saying 'you have to have faith, people like Benny Hinn pray for people.' These opinions may be the result of her apparent lack of experience of spiritual healing in her own church although she believes that media personalities such as Benny Hinn, a media preacher and healer, are more successful in their prayer for healing. On the other hand she may not have wanted me to be delving into the activities of her church and aimed to protect the people with whom she worships.

Prayer and faith are closely linked as indicate by Respondent 3 below

Respondent 3 (URC): *Now, gifts of healing do not operate in isolation from other gifts of the Holy Spirit. You will almost certainly need to operate gifts of faith, whilst working the gifts of healing*
This is also stated in 1 Corinthians 12. If a person, for example have a cancer, which could be terminal, they would need to get the word of God for their situation, they would need to know for certainty in their own heart what God is saying to them, that he will for example, carry them through and the prayers may need to have the same—and you may find that you need a gift of miraculous powers to go with that healing as well
You will certainly need to be used by God in the Gifts of the Holy Spirit that has to be with the mind of God. You will need the mind of God's wisdom, to know how and when to pray, the mind of God's Knowledge to know what to pray for and the mind of God's discernment and knowledge in discernment are vital.
For example, when praying for cancers it is perfectly valid if the Lord lays it on you to command the cancer to 'DIE' in the Name of Jesus and to 'condemn' in the Name of Jesus. The implication is that the cancer is some form of demonic force and you would be amazed how often it works, but you must know from the Lord whether that is the way to pray or not.

There are many instances in the gospels where Jesus healed the sick and there is evidence that Respondent 3 believes in the power of the Holy

Spirit and the influence of faith. In John 5 the man who was healed at the pool of Bethesda was there because he believed in the power of the Holy Spirit as he waited for someone to allow or help him to get into the pool that was stirred up by the angel. The interview with Respondent 10 given in section 6.3 above also indicates some evidence of healing through prayer, and indicates how knowledge "gained through discernment" is understood.

Although Robert et al. (2009) state that no research has successfully attempted to measure the psychological effects of intercessory prayer, for Respondent 10 the psychological effect of knowing her baby was now growing normally and the stunted growth in her uterus had been reversed must have appeared miraculous to someone who believes in prayer for healing. The apparent intercessory prayer and discerning spirit of the visiting minister may have strengthened her faith in the fact that God works through appointed and anointed people. Moreover, it must have appeared miraculous to her that the minister could discern her needs although she was not overtly presenting her own needs but was presenting her sister's needs. Maybe she thought her own needs were less important than her sister's as her sister's needs were in an emergency critical situation.

Prayer for Healing for Specific Illnesses

During intercessory prayer, which is a core part of the order of service in URC the healer may pray for healing of a specific condition, as illustrated in the extract from Respondent 3 in the previous section.

Sometimes prayers are said for specific conditions and other times prayers are said for the healing of the whole person. It may be the healer who asks the person for specifics when they request prayer or it may be the person requesting the prayer that offers to tell the healer what they would like him to pray about. In the URC the healer often asks for this information. The COGIC members are more reluctant to offer information to the healer and appear to prefer it when the healer tells them what he thinks the problem is.

Respondent 6, (URC) makes reference to prayer for healing of specific conditions.

Respondent 6 (URC) The chiropractor assesses my pain and explains what they are doing. The people who pray for me know about my pain. I would not go to a spiritual healer who knows nothing about me.
Interviewer: 'Is it cured now?
Respondent: 'I have to be careful' (reticent answer)

This respondent believed that she needed a specialist in back problems and she also needed the spiritual healer to pray for her specific problem. She did not receive a miracle but believed that healing was ongoing. She also had to take some responsibility in seeking and securing on-going healing 'I have to be careful.' There is an indication here that although she clearly had a condition that required 'medical' attention she could not adopt the sick role to be excluded from all her responsibilities and part of that responsibility is to actively seek treatment or a cure for the illness.

It could be argued that prayer can encourage or discourage people to adopt or reject the sick role. If they are engaging in health seeking behaviour whilst continuing with their day to day activities in the belief that seeking prayer will result in healing, they may follow the pattern of actions set out in Zola's (1973) typology to seek medical care at the same time that they are seeking prayer. They may also choose self treatment and prayer as in Dingwall's (1976) 'Illness Action Model.'

Respondent 6 did not excuse herself from her day to day activities whilst she consulted with the chiropractor and used the same approach when seeking spiritual healing. She did not adopt the sick role that Parsons (1975) describes in his 1951 model discussed in Chapter 2, without taking some positive steps first to make herself better. By adopting the sick role she could have got some sympathy from friends, family and work colleagues. They would find it easier to accept that she could not function fully in some tasks, such as lifting and carrying, although she could continue to perform other tasks unaffected by her specific back problem.

There are similarities between respondent 2's account of prayer for healing with how the participants in the study of Hawley and Irurita (1998) describe their pain and discomfort and how they sought comfort from God through prayer.

Respondent 2: *(URC) 'yesterday I had a cough and I was taking cough mixture. I thought I would not be able to come to church today. I was going to buy some cough mixture, but I thought I would be late for church so I came straight to church. As the service proceeded, I prayed and asked God to heal my cough and I stopped coughing.'*

The study of Hawley and Irurita (1998) on prayer in nursing found respondents focusing prayer on the situation at the time by using words such as 'Lord calm this apprehension' when they were feeling apprehensive. According to Hawley and Irurita this is prayer for survival rather than instinctive prayer where the person without thinking cries for help when they may only be able to speak one or two sentences.

Although the prayers in the URC are usually said by the minister, Respondent 2 did not request prayer from the minister but prayed quietly, probably in one or more sentences and she was able to focus on a specific need. Like respondent 10 quoted at length in section 6.3 above, she appears to be able to pray for specific need for herself or for others.

Respondent 10 explained her use of prayer as well as the medical (drug) approach to claiming her healing but clearly believed that healing of her sore throat was through prayer and touch directed by a force from outside and that she was used as the channel for her own healing.

Distance Healing versus Contact Healing

The evidence from this study suggests that the respondents believe the practice of prayer for people at a distance has some effect although the effect may be as beneficial to the sender of the prayer as the receiver.

Neither O'Laoire (1997) or Shlitz and Braud (1997) study addressed the spiritual aspect of prayer. As noted in Chapter 2, scientific research that has attempted to measure the effectiveness of prayer and healing has focused on psychological experiments rather than a spiritual approach. This may be because explaining the spiritual aspect cannot be demonstrated by psychological experiments and remains a mystery and will remain a mystery to the human understanding. This understanding is equally clouded in contrasting the two churches on focused prayer as no explanation from observations or interviews was offered about **how** prayer works. There were statements and activities such as outlined in the observations extracts below that support their experiences that when they prayed for healing or when someone prayed for them there was some lessening of their feelings of discomfort or disease.

Prayer for distant healing takes place in every COGIC service on request, or simply for members who are absent from the service and who have requested or had prayers requested on their behalf. The URC focused prayer is directed by the minister who selects appointed elders to assist him in the laying of hands during healing services. In the URC prayer for distant healing take place every Sunday and healing services are focused in the fifth Sunday of the month.

Prayer meeting 1: COGIC
COGIC has a session that is focused on prayer or prayer meeting where members of the church meet and are asked to pray. This meeting is not always led by the minister. The pastor may delegate the leading role to a well trusted church member such as an elder, deacon or 'mother'. Older female members are afforded the title of 'mother' as recognition of their long service of commitment to attend service, pray with younger members and also provide support for church members including the Pastor. This focused prayer may also take place during a divine or other service 'under the direction of the Holy Spirit' and at the request of a trusted member.
The prayer meeting is moderated by someone chosen by the Pastor. The Pastor directs the moderator (or mother) by specifying the scripture to be read and the focus of the prayer meeting. The prayer meeting opens with a prayer song from the Redemption Songs hymn book. A scripture reading and another song follow this. A member of the congregation hands prayer cushions to others in the meeting. The 'service' is then handed back to the Pastor, who states that the prayer meeting should focus on a series of meetings over the Easter weekend. At the prayer meeting attenders kneeled and prayed a Pentecostal prayer where each person prays their own prayer, but everyone prays at the same time. This continued for about 30 minutes. The Pastor then asked one person to pray, to conclude this section of the meeting. A song and the closing prayer by the pastor follows this and the 'benediction' (Now may the saving Grace of our Lord and Saviour Jesus Christ, rest remain and abide with us all), is repeated by everyone present.

Dr. Gwen Rose

A greeting to 'welcome' me and one or two members of the prayer meeting followed this.
This greeting felt distanced. There was no real warmth. Any warmth was superficial although probably someone outside the 'faith' would view this as a warm welcome.

Prayer meeting 2 COGIC
'The moderator gave n introductory speech of encouragement about the Christian faith and why we should pray, to the group. I was offered a hymnbook, but no bible this time.
A Pentecostal prayer where everyone prays at the same time, but prays their own individual prayer was offered as a means of dedication of the service.
The service continued with the singing of Hymn 325 from the Redemption Songs hymnbook. This was followed by a session of loud and articulated praise and worship.
This was followed by another session of Pentecostal prayer. Each person adopted a different prayer position such as kneeling or sitting. The moderator stood for this prayer session. Following this session there was a general praise and worship session during which one member of the group became very animated, shouting praises. Some members spoke in tongues and another member began to rebuke the devil in English.

Those who attend prayer meetings regularly include particularly the older women members of the church. The prayer meetings have a similar format to the services on Sunday except that the emphasis is on prayer. The recorded observation of both services illustrates the similarities in the format and structure of the services.

Although prayers for healing are said in different ways and at different times in both churches, there is always a time when praying is the focus of the service. The prayer meeting in COGIC places the emphasis on prayer for many different things including healing, whereas in the URC services there is a separate focus on healing apart from general prayer.

Healing service in the URC
The session starts with a period of quiet time for reflective contemplation.
Song 22 from Songs of Fellowship;

Invitation by the minister to join the healing service and to come forward for the laying of hands and prayer;
The presiding minister invited another minister to join him at this time. Before the start of the main service, they had prepared together for this part of the service through discussion and prayer.
The second minister went forward and they prayed quietly together whilst the congregation looked on and joined quietly in prayer if they so wished.
The organist played quiet background music throughout the healing service. Seven members of the congregation went forward for prayer and laying on of hands. Initially two people went forward and each of them was prayed for individually by the ministers both laying hands on each person and praying.
The other members went forward and each person was prayed for individually.
The seventh person was in tears and was comforted by another member of the congregation and then one of the elders. This member was comforted for some time after the services was closed.
The service closed with the minister inviting the whole congregation to join in holding hands and the minister prayed. This was different and the first time I observed this approach in this church.
The final song was a joyful one: 148.
The benediction of the Grace was then said: may the grace of—

Differences in How Prayer is Administered in the Churches

Prayer for healing takes place in both churches but each church take a different approach. The Pentecostals such as COGIC pray according to the leading of the Holy Spirit and not according to a preset routine or a pre-written prayer. Any appointed minister can be asked to pray for the healing of an individual and at any time during the service. The altar call for prayer does not specify requests only for healing prayer, but also for receiving the Baptism of the Holy Spirit, prayer for repentance or consecration or prayer for forgiveness of sins. The URC prayers for healing are conducted in a routine manner (see examples of healing service in URC in Chapter 4. Not all the ministers pray for healing during the service but all ministers pray for forgiveness of sins during the service. There is a healing service in the URC every 5th Sunday of the month however, there is no specific healing service in the COGIC.

Dr. Gwen Rose

Much of the healing ministry of the URC observed in this study is similar to the practices described more than a decade ago by Lucas (1997) in his book on Christian healing in Anglo-Catholic churches. The URC like the Anglicans use a ritualistic approach to prayer for healing. The intercessory prayer in the weekly Sunday services includes prayer for those who are sick in hospital and at home (see orders of service in chapter 4). The healing services also include focused prayer for healing. In COGIC, prayer for healing is ad-hoc and unorganized, this is the result of the Pentecostal belief in spontaneous prompting of the Holy Spirit to pray for specific situations.

Lucas does not explicitly contrast ritualistic approaches with the Pentecostal style of services for prayer and healing. He believes that it is wise to choose a method to conduct healing services which acknowledges that people respond to familiar rituals. People may, however, also respond favourably to change in rituals if the purpose is explained and there is a good reason for the change. For example if there is a well known healer or minister with a different approach people often welcome the change especially if the results are positive and identified in reports of testimonies of healing.

Both COGIC and URC, however, accompany prayer for healing with the 'laying on of hands' and both churches may hold hands and pray as a team during the service. The URC ministers pray alone, with the leadership team members and the congregation in silent agreement, whilst COGIC will pray in Pentecostal style where the leadership team or the whole congregation prays together at the same time to illustrate their understanding of the down pouring of the Holy Spirit at Pentecost.

In the URC, music and songs are chosen before the service and these are sung at appropriate places in the order of the service. A musician may choose a prayer song or refrain that is appropriate at the time. During the 'laying on of hands' (therapeutic touch) there may be an appropriate refrain that has been chosen before the service or may be chosen at the beginning of the laying of hands by the musician who is in tune with the spirit of the service. In COGIC the songs, except those scheduled for the choir or the young people's group, are also chosen in an unorganized way under the 'leading of the Hoy Spirit' as exemplified in the prayer meetings at COGIC reported in this chapter.

Lucas gives accounts of liturgical healing services and non-liturgical healing (formal and informal) services which are similar to the URC services where the services include an invitation or call to worship, thanksgiving and praise, prayers of intercession, readings, silence an address or sermon, confession, laying on of hands and sometimes anointing with oil, absolution, the Lord's prayer and a final blessing. There is a similar framework for the services in COGIC although this may not be adhered to in preference to the spontaneous prompts under the leading of the Holy Spirit.

The non-liturgical service in the URC is a simple framework involving hymns and songs, a talk, confession of sins, a declaration of forgiveness and intercessory prayer for the sick who are not present in the service. The intercessory prayer for the sick may take the form of prayer for the person directly or through another person who represents that person during the prayer. During prayer the elders and volunteers from the congregation may form a circle and lay hands on a member of the congregation who has requested healing. They may also form a circle where a chair is placed in the middle of the circle and the member requesting prayer for another person sits in the chair in the middle as representing the person who is not present in the service. The same ritual is performed for those who are present and requests prayer for healing. The leader will conclude the prayer by saying 'We pray for X'. After a time of silence the leader says 'Thank you Lord' and this may be followed with a time of prayer for others where their names and location are called out (for example, 'John in Cambridge.') There is a pause followed by 'Thank you Lord'.

The method and processes of closing the service in both churches usually include a final attempt to offer prayer for healing which may mention the need for healing from suffering which people may not have announced, or been recognized by others.

The minister or the moderator invites the congregation to say the grace to each other or whilst facing each other. This provides an opportunity to seek forgiveness from each other and to offer words that encourage healing, to each other. In the URC these words are said at the end of the service whilst making eye contact with other members of the congregation.

'*May the Grace of God, the Father, Son and Holy Spirit be with you now and forever Amen.*' Those words are said to each individual with a hand-shake. '*Peace be with you*', and may be said during the service at a point selected by the minister or at the end of the service again as decided by the minister.

In COGIC these words are said together as a prayer (but not to each other with handshakes as in the URC.) '*And now may the Saving Grace of our Lord and Saviour Jesus Christ be with you now and forever. Amen.*' COGIC do not say the 'Peace.' As an alternative, the 'Benediction' may be said as an indication that the service has come to a close and as a final prayer of thanks to God and blessing for the congregation. In COGIC the minister or moderator may ask a church member (usually an officer) to say the benediction whilst in URC it is likely to be the minister who says the final blessing.

In the URC the Grace is usually said at the beginning of the service and the Peace is said during or at the end of the service when the congregation is invited to participate. Both formulae are said by everyone to each other. Each person repeats the words as they look around the congregation with a smile. It is important that there is eye contact with some members of the congregation when the grace is being said. The instruction is that the grace is said to each other. It is therefore not explained why some members of the congregation may say the grace with their eyes closed. What is more bizarre is where members of the congregation say the peace or the grace to someone that they are in conflict with and continue the conflict, as explained in the section on dispute and fission in chapter 5.

The minister of the URC says the prayer of forgiveness and with his authority says the sins of the congregation have been forgiven, yet members of congregation may not be able to accept this statement of forgiveness. In COGIC, forgiveness is not declared by the minister; people can only seek forgiveness and 'healing' through their own atonement with God by genuinely repenting of their sin.

This approach is less likely to encourage individual forgiveness and healing, although the forgiveness approach to the ritual of confession that is practised by the Catholic priests may have a similar effect for those who believe that the minister can declare forgiveness.

The doctrine of COGIC does not teach the members to accept that the minister can declare forgiveness. They believe that forgiveness can only be granted by God after confession of sins to God.

Conclusion

This chapter examined the processes of seeking health through the use of supplicative and intercessory prayer, using the health belief and health promotion models. It goes beyond the earlier work of Byrd (1998) and Dossey (1997) and other work examined in the most recent survey of how outcomes might be affected by prayer by Narayansamy and Narayansamy (2008), in that it does not treat prayer as a simple undifferentiated variable, but examines it as a complex and variegated social process. Like Narayansamy and Narayansamy, however, this thesis points to prayer as complementary to professional healthcare in allowing the body to heal, triggering mechanism for counteracting stress, and promoting positive emotions, activating the hormonal and cardiovascular system, and evoking psychological responses such as decreased heart rate and decreased blood pressure.

Chapter Five

Laying on of Hands

Introduction

This chapter examines the concept 'laying on of hands' as an approach to using touch as technique in spiritual healing. Laying on of hands (LH) is one of the three activities (along with prayer and music) observed during the data collection for this study which can be analysed in terms of the theory of health promotion. Like prayer it is a specific activity which can be measured in terms of how many times this is done, which in principle suggests we could carry out outcome studies on how many times it is successful. However it is difficult to assess its effects in isolation as it operates in conjunction with prayer, faith and music. It is also somewhat arbitrary to differentiate between the therapeutic touch in a non-religious context and the laying on of hands. In the medical/nursing field touch is often used a healing gesture especially for patients with skin conditions and patients who believe they are contagious or wretched. Touch provides a human to human contact and is reassuring to the person receiving the gesture of touch in a therapeutic/healing situation. It indicates that another person, the healer cares. Therapeutic touch has always been a medical/nursing skill that contributes to the healing. For example when a patient has extensive eczema or HIV or AIDS, the doctor or nurse may make a point of touching the patient to reassure them that their condition is not contagious.

This chapter was born out of observations of church services and healing services in both churches and the outcome of interrogating the data. Laying on of hands will be shown to be capable of being analysed as a health promotion activity within the administration of spiritual healing, and outside it in alternative complementary therapies such as massage therapy, demonstrating care and compassion. This activity takes place in an organized way in the URC whilst in COGIC it takes place in an unstructured way as the fieldwork data reported below shows, which demonstrates the contrast noted throughout this research that, Belcher et al. (2001) note for this activity, that in most Pentecostal churches it is impossible to separate a theology of healing from the life of the church.

It will be noted that reports about the 'laying on of hands' and anointing with oil from the respondents and from observation during the administration of spiritual healing indicated some similarities with therapeutic touch administered during medical and nursing examinations, osteopathy, physiotherapy and massage therapy.

Definitions and Use of the Terms within the Clinical and Popular Literatures

In the discussion of the clinical and popular literature (Lambert et al. 2008, Krieger 1975, Krieger et al 1979, Barlow et al 2008) showed the closeness of Christian understandings of the laying on of hands from biblical times to the present concept of therapeutic touch, actually defined by Krieger (1975) as consisting of "the simple placing of hands for about 10-15 minutes on or close to the body of an ill person by someone who intends to help of heal the person." Hallett's (2004) case study treats therapeutic touch and laying on of hands as more or less the same thing.

Section 1 thus showed that the clinical literature tends to define Therapeutic Touch rather loosely, as an interaction where there is direct or indirect contact between the healer and the patient with direct contact not being necessary. Indeed they may include all the occasions where the doctor touches, prods or taps the patient during conventional diagnostic procedures.[2] It can be anything from massage therapy and acupuncture

---

[2] All medical and nursing requires technical skills that include look, listen, and feel (touch) as outlined in Hunter (2008). Hunter describes an example in the technical skills of touch in respiratory assessment of a patient as 'feel that the chest movements are symmetrical. Chest expansion can be observed or

to anointing with oil as recommended in the bible and practised in the churches. This contrasts with some of the non-clinical popular literature such as King (1976) and Lawrence (2001) who distinguish sharply between contact healing and non-contact healing

In both direct and indirect contact, therapeutic touch is an interaction with the personal space of the person receiving healing by the person giving healing. Although Sayre-Adams et al.'s (1995) textbook does not require therapeutic touch to be performed in a specific physical context; they assert the person performing the act of touch is in a meditative state that is similar to that of prayer and meditation. It has even been hypothesized by Achterberg (1985:120) that the physical effects of this mental state may be the result of the neurological processes involved in imagining or thinking about healing and suggests it is "the inter-relatedness among neurons and their activities that is critical to the assumption that imagery serves an integrative mechanism between the mental and physical processes". If the healers and the recipients conceive that every living thing has an energy field, most illness has started before developing into a physical illness. Then the touch takes place when the energy field of the healer touches the energy field of the person seeking healing (Krieger 1975). Stony Brook University Medical Centre provides an example of a hospital website (http://www.stonybrookmedicalcenter.org/) that systematically recommends such ideas to its patients. Within such discourses it is a small step to suggest that the life-giving breath of God described in the first chapter of Genesis can play a similar role.

The discussions of cardiac treatment on the Stony Brook website fall in with this imagery of Therapeutic Touch as a type of energy medicine where the therapist moves his hands over the patient's energy field, extending the concept of medicine beyond that of some kind of liquid or solid substance that is taken into the body in some form through the skin, mouth or nose to anything which has healing properties if it is the correct medicine for the individual or the illness. Therapeutic touch, however, does not quite

---

felt to determine the depth and quality of movement of the chest during both inspiration and expiration' No one asserts that the spiritual healer requires the same level of technical skills as described by Hunter (2008).

fit into the conventional idea of medicine as the 'substance' transferred into the body is not tangible and cannot be measured.

Laying on of hands, along with anointing with oil, as described in the bible is a healing ritual of the Jewish tradition. The Jerome Bible Commentary (Brown et al 1996) and Lucas (1997) describe how this is incorporated as part of the broad ministry of healing in the early church, as described in James, 5, where the apostle bids 'if there is any sick among you let him call the elders to pray over him and anoint him with oil'. Rice (2001) confirms that the early church as well as the church today has continued the practice of healing using both the spoken word and touch, as accounts in the book of Acts and the gospels indicate. James 5 makes the connection between healing and the use of anointing oil.

Harvey (2004) postulates that James 5 gives us a glimpse of the early church, the Jewish sect who practised both the art of medicine and spiritual healing. Mark 7, Mark 6 and John 9 also make reference to touch and the use of oil in healing. Interestingly, the only gospel that does not mention this healing model and process is Luke who was a physician. Spiritual healing by 'laying on of hands' is not determined by a time factor and passages such as James 5 are not specific about a time factor or the method that the elders should use in 'laying hands on the sick'. There are different approaches to using touch as healing techniques in spiritual healing, but Lambert (2008) show how much in common the biblical spiritual healing through laying on of hands appears to have with the definitions of therapeutic touch in the literature just cited and assert "Proximal Spiritual Healing is commonly termed Laying on of hands and include therapeutic touch." Graham (1999) asserts that laying on of hands has similar properties to Reiki and other oriental healing traditions in that it uses the universal life energy as the formula for healing.

Within the bible, healing by the laying on hands is seen uncomplicatedly as miraculous; but we need to ask whether this understanding of "miracles" in biblical texts involves the same sense of scientific inexplicability as today, when people in the bible did not have the same understanding of science. Some biblical examples of 'miracles' using laying on of hands (touch) for healing are: The woman with the issue of blood in Mark, Peter and John at the Gate Beautiful when the man who has been lame from birth was healed and immediately started to walk (run) in Acts, Elijah, when he raised the dead son of the widow in 1 Kings and Moses when he stretched out his rod and the dead sea was separated for the safe crossing of the Israelites and the destruction of the Egyptians in Exodus 14. These are seen as miraculous happenings that did not involve direct touch. Obviously anything at all which happens has proximate physical causes, and equally anything which happens, for a Christian happens within the creative will of God, and it is common ground that phenomena which once seemed inexplicable, such as lightning, are now well understood in terms of proximate physical causes.

For those who reject traditional Christian discourse, this can mean that lightning can be seen as less, or not at all miraculous, and that all the miracles of the bible should be seen as either, like lightning, as having normal proximate physical causes or as not to have happened in the way reported in the bible. For these, the depiction of these "miraculous" events is part of a pre-modern mythological world view that makes assumptions about divine reality and intervention which might no longer be tenable. Some religious people over the last couple of centuries have turned this argument on its head, and insist that genuine miracles are not just things which are inexplicable right now because we do not know enough about God's creation, but are necessarily inexplicable except as direct interventions by God without any other proximate cause, physical or otherwise, and which are supernatural without at the same time being un-natural. Whether the concept of creative action, which is outside or beyond the nature of creation, is philosophically coherent, remains a matter for debate which is beyond the scope of this thesis. Christians and Christian scholarship are thus divided on the question of whether or not miracles have happened in the past and whether or not they happen today. The issue is not about whether or not the bible is accepted, but also about how it is interpreted.

The Practice of Laying on of hands or Therapeutic Touch

Both churches practise the laying on of hands for healing according to what they see as a biblical pattern, where the elders are called upon to lay hands on the sick (James 5). The ritual is practiced in the services by the ministers and other appointed healers, approved by the ministers. Direct touch or laying on of hands was observed as a regular practice. It resembled the practices recorded in both the clinical literature by observers like Hallett (2004) who describes practitioners moving their hands in a downwards motion, a few inches from the body of the recipient and in popular literature such as by Lawrence (2001:120-121), a practising healer who describes the energy field as the aura.

The observations and interviews showed that the services in COGIC were not structured as healing services. 'Laying on of hands' took different forms, using different methods such as placing the hand on the forehead, or a position where there is pain, such as the back, the knee, or the abdomen. The same approach was used in the URC although it took place in special healing services and the rituals were more focused. The Pentecostal church does not have a structured and organized method of 'laying on of hands' whereas the URC church has a regular healing service every 5th Sunday of the month where church attendees are invited to the ritualistic activity of healing prayer accompanied by the 'laying on of hands' by the minister. In the observations in both churches there were instances when oil was used to anoint those requesting healing.

Both congregations, however, draw deeply on biblical narratives of healing. For example, this extract from observation of a healing service in the URC illustrates calling on the elders to use laying on of hands to heal:

The healing session starts with healing by laying on of hands (touch) for one of the elders who moved forward for healing.
The minister prayed and the other elders agreed with him in prayer. Each of the four elders and the minister laid hands on each member of the congregation who moved forward for healing.(one elder per member of the congregation) The minister also laid hands on the forehead of each person who requested prayer. The first two persons who came forward had two people laying hands o on them for healing, the minister and an elder.
Then the pattern changed. The minister laid hands on the shoulders of the second person. The elders supported by resting their hands on the back and the hands of the person.
For the 3rd person the minister held her hands and moved to a more quiet prayer.

The 4th person had similar treatment (Hands of the minister on her shoulder, then on her forehead as the minister engaged in quiet but intensive prayer.
5th request: The minister placed his hands on her shoulders as she verbalized her request.
The organist played a song 'Such Love' quietly as background music throughout the healing service.

Here the responding is implicitly drawing on James 5 and narratives at the beginning of Acts which include both the first healing miracles by the disciples, and the clearest description of speaking in tongues. Acts 3 narrates the story of Peter healing the lame man, where he made it clear to the man that he did not have money to give him as he expected. Peter made sure that the man was prepared to receive and then 'laid hands on him'. Although not what he expected (money) because he expected to receive something, an environment for healing was created. Peter took the man who had never walked 'by the right hand and lifted him up and his feet and ankle bones received strength.' But, as Respondent 2 emphasizes, it is not necessarily the laying on of hands that brings healing; it may be the miraculous working of prayer through the Holy Spirit.

Neither church routinely seeks miraculous healing, although occasionally there may be a visiting speaker in COGIC who will attempt to practise healing in the way Peter did in Acts 3. The church members do not assume, however, that this was the regular pattern and process of healing that Peter conducted. They may, however, carry out laying on of hands and at times, anointing the affected area or the person's head with oil, without expecting immediate healing but assuming long-term benefit. This does fit into the model of health seeking behaviour or health promotion activity as described by Ewles and Simnett (2003). For example we may consider the rest of the notes of observation of the healing service in the URC quoted above:

Healing service A
Then there was the call for volunteers to receive healing through the laying on of hands. The preacher then recalled his experience of a service where he said 'someone in the meeting has a problem from very early age and this is to do with forgiveness. After the service a young man came to him and confessed he fell out with his mother at a very young age and had never forgiven her.'

This session then took a different approach where the volunteers were asked to show their hands and the ministers would come to them in the congregation and lay hands on them and pray.
The congregation was invited to raise their hand, point to the prayer team and the volunteer and pray with them. The musician was asked to play the song 'Be still and know that I am God', No. 40 from the hymn book.
The church elders were invited to join the minister in the laying on of hands for healing.
The elders engaged in a group prayer and joining hands with the minister before the laying on of hands ceremony. The elders were identified by their response to the invitation by the minister to join him for the healing service.
The minister also invited the rest of the congregation to participate by stretching their hands towards those who requested healing. There were six requests in total; three at the initial invitation.
The healing session started with healing . . . [notes quoted above on previous page] . . . . The organist played a song, 'Such Love' quietly as background music throughout the healing service.
The healing service now focused on those receiving healing and those delivering healing whilst the rest of the congregation watched (and probably prayed).
One or two members of the congregation joined in by stretching their hands forward as requested by the minister.
When all the prayer requests had been addressed the elders moved quickly from the laying on of hands to a group prayer.
Members of the congregation who needed help to go for prayer were helped by members of the congregation and escorted back to their seats after the healing ceremony.
The service closed with a prayer by the minister and a blessing for the congregation.
This was followed by a short time for silent individual prayer as the organist played a musical rendition.

Healing service B: URC
Reflective time for the congregation
Song 22 from the Songs of Fellowship
Invitation by the minister to join the healing service and to come forward for the laying on of hands and prayer

The presiding minister invited another minister to join him at this time. Before the start of the main service, they had prepared together for this part of the service through discussion and prayer.
The second minister went forward and they prayed quietly together whilst the congregation looked on and joined quietly in prayer if they so wished.
The organist played quiet background music throughout the healing service, 7 members of the congregation went forward for prayer and laying on of hands. Initially two people went forward and each of them was prayed for individually by the ministers both laying hands on each person and prayed.
The other members went forward and each person was prayed for individually.
The seventh person was in tears and was comforted by another member of the congregation and then one of the elders. This member was comforted for some time after the services was closed.
The service closed with the minister inviting the whole congregation to join in holding hands and the minister prayed. This was different and the first time I observed this approach in this church.
The final song was a joyful one: 148
The benediction and the Grace were said by the minister as the closing and dismissal prayer.

These two extracts illustrate a different approach by different ministers to the specified healing services in URC. In the first extract the minister relays his own experience of administering healing through discernment. Maybe this was to encourage confidence in his ability to administer healing to members of the congregation. He invited audience participation by asking them to raise their hands to the person requesting healing. The service closed with silence accompanied by meditative music. In the second extract the service starts with reflection and meditation and did not directly invite 'audience' participation. The service did, however, adopt the style of laying on of hands by the church elders as stated in 1 Timothy 4.

We may contrast the URC service with the observation of a COGIC service (at a convention):

At the beginning of the prayer session the minister stated that all unwelcome spirits would be banished from the church. This included spirits from the past. She related an incident about a swarm of wasps that had housed themselves in the 'vestry'. She implied that a member of the church was encouraging the swarm of wasps. She was adamant that the wasps (by fumigation if necessary) had to go and if the member had difficulties with this, he/she would also have to go.

Unlike other COGIC services, an invitation was extended to the congregation to come forward for prayer for healing especially if they had any unwelcome spirit in themselves or their family. 95% of the congregation of about 250 formed a line to receive healing. Each person had individual prayer and was anointed with olive oil by the healer (minister) In the background was a group of singers who sang the same prayer song throughout the healing session

The picture filled with animated activities. There were people falling to the floor, people who were dancing, people who were laughing, crying and the healer danced with them, cried with them. If they fell to the floor, her assistants helped those who were on the floor and continued to pray with them. She named the spirits that she was praying about. Some of these were disobedience, stubbornness, fear, anger and unbelief. She stood on a chair whilst she prayed for some of the 'patients' One person received the baptism of the Holy Spirit and another person surrendered their life to God as announced by the 'healer.'

Before this service, a protective prayer was offered so that the healer was not afflicted by the condition of the person to whom they were administering healing. During a service, the minister may ask the congregation to support his prayers by stretching out their hands during the prayer for healing. This is a means of engaging those who wish to contribute to the process and actively participate in prayer. This part of the service usually follows on from the usual service where the energy field in the church is charged with God's (Good) energy and the majority of the people are feeling uplifted from the prayer, singing, music, sermon and the testimonies of encouragement.

Individual Experiences of Laying on of Hands

Individual respondents may use their religious framework for the understanding of healing to interpret secular therapies. The extract from COGIC Respondent 1 below describes her experience of using prayer to get the most out of massage in the healing process.

I was feeling unwell and went for a massage. This was done with soft music in the background and the masseur used different oils. I was also praying diligently for healing. I started to cough blood and what looked like bits of my lung. After this episode of coughing I felt better. When I went to see the doctor later, I was told that the blood did not come from my lungs. However he ordered a scan of my lungs. The results of the scan showed recent scar tissues on my lungs and the doctor confirmed that the blood and what appeared to be bits of my lungs were very likely to be from the scars that showed on the scan.

In this respondent's' account, and also that of respondent 5 above, where conditions had already been diagnosed by a medical doctor, prayer was accompanied with touch and the anointing of oil. It appears that in both scenarios the doctors were able to confirm healing which may or may not have been spiritual healing. Respondent 1 was told by the doctor that there was recent scar tissue on her lungs which contradicted his earlier statement prior to the scan that the blood did not come from her lungs. Respondent 5 returned to the doctor for confirmation of her illness (or her healing) and did not have to take the medication prescribed by the doctor.

In the extracts from the respondents and my observations there is no example of touch purely by itself accomplishing healing. All the 'Laying on of hands' activities that were observed in the healing services were accompanied by prayer and sometimes music.
Those healed often describe improvement in their state of health as feelings of calmness, reduced pain, lifting of anxiety, improvement in conditions of feeling ill, a feeling of walking on air after the 'treatment'. It was also often reported that after massage therapy there is a general feeling of euphoria. Sometimes listening to the person seeking healing followed by a gentle touch on the arm, shoulder or forehead at the 'right time' could have a long lasting effect. Therapeutic touch, where the professional or the healer touches the person with a health seeking request, invokes a certain amount of trust. In such relationships where the person seeking healing feels they are not alone, they become less anxious and tense where reduced tension of the muscles reduces pain. This is illustrated in the first observation of a URC healing service described under the heading 'healing service A' in section chapter 4 section.3.

During massage therapy the body is relaxed, the lymphatic system functions more efficiently in removing chemicals from the blood stream. This is similar to the body's response to physical activity or exercise. After massage therapy, the client is usually advised to drink water to flush the toxins. The many beneficial effects of massage therapy is outlined in Moyer's (2004) meta-analysis of massage therapy research. This paper explains that when compared to the medical model of treatments, there are limitations but there is a psychotherapy perspective on mood enhancing effects. It may be that the body has a similar response when spiritual healing is administered whether by direct contact (using the healer) or indirect contact (participating in a church service or receiving distant prayer).

The spiritual healer may intuitively 'feel' the person's pain through transference and empathy (Rogers 1990, Fleischman1990) and the physical process of reaching out to the person confirm a psychological spiritual process. This is also sensed and the person may receive or reject the healing energy. Rogers suggests that it is the attitude and the tone of the healer (counsellor) that encourages the client to accept a diagnosis of client's feelings. In spiritual healing, using touch as part of the therapy implies that the attitude of the healer is intended to be empathetic and the person will receive it as such. The healer is advised not to 'lay hands on anyone hastily and to keep yourself pure'. The spiritual healer may not understand the chemical requirements of the body and may fail to give the recipient appropriate advice. Equally it may be that the miraculous or mysterious effect of spiritual healing allows healing to take place regardless of how the healer or the healed behave.

Below are brief parts of extracts previously cited from respondents in response to the question from the interviewer *"Have you administered spiritual healing to anyone?"* These extracts also illustrate a certain level of trust in the respondent from her friend.

Respondent 11 COGIC
Respondent: Oh! A friend of mine came here one day and said the uncle was very ill he was rushed to hospital. He had a mild stroke—He was in pain so I said 'Let us go and see him'. So we went and he was crawling, he was in so much pain. I did not go with the intention of praying for him but just before we left 'I felt something say, pray for him' So I asked 'Would you mind if I pray for you? He said he did not mind. So I just prayed. I laid my hand on him and

Dr. Gwen Rose

prayed and he started dancing. It was so instant that I was surprised myself. I don't understand how these things work.

Note the words: *'I did not go with the intention of praying for him.'*

What was it that moved her to pray and lay hands on the sick person? It could be seen as a prompting of the Holy Spirit, a movement of compassion or an attempt to practise her belief and faith in the healing powers that has been invested in her as a person and a practising Christian. The resulting effect must have been rewarding and reinforced the initial motivation to visit someone who is ill.

Respondent 8, a COGIC member, makes reference to instances when she believed healing had taken place through her own touch and where she believed that 'God was speaking to her directly'. Not these words from the interview cited at much greater length 3 above.

'I felt that these words were God speaking to me directly and at the invitation for prayer I went forward for prayer. This is not something that I do lightly or on a regular basis. As I stood at the altar I started to pray and I was playing with my throat, like this! using my hands to gently touch and rub my throat (as she said this she was demonstrating her actions of rubbing her throat during her prayer)' I felt that something had moved in my throat but I did not say anything to anyone.

She believed that by massaging her throat and praying for herself she was able to claim healing. Rubbing her throat and praying drew from the energy field of prayer and with the energy generated from her own altered state of consciousness, she was able to self heal. This action was probably not predetermined and her explanation would probably be that it was the inspiration of the Holy Spirit during her openness to receive healing. The environment of worship and music was also a contributory factor. She may have been influenced by non-academic popular healing literature like Lawrence (2001) who suggests that actions such as placing the palms of the hand together holds positive energy within. Where this person would normally be laying hands on another person she used the same energy to heal herself. She described the result as 'I felt something had moved in my throat.'

Below is a description of the apparently 'forceful' touching action of the minister during a service at the COGIC convention. The most outstanding aspect of this service was when the speaker came to a young lady who was sitting in the row of seats in front of me.

He came to her, held her by the hand and said 'I have been directed by the spirit to pray for you' He then led her to the front of the audience and said to her' You have double trouble' Am I right? She nodded in agreement. He then said 'The Lord tell me to tell you that' 'You will come through and you will be stronger' He then proceeded to pray for her, Before he started to pray for her two senior members of the congregation (one male and one female who was the Bishop's wife as she was introduced as such earlier in the service) came and stood behind the lady. As he prayed for her, he laid his right hand on her forehead and with what appeared to be slightly forceful action or gentle push, she fell backwards. She was prevented from falling directly by the supporting 'ministers' who supported her on to the floor as she fell backwards. The speaker continued to address the congregation.

My observation possibilities at this point were rather limited as I could not see clearly what was happening from where I was sitting. The lady did not stay for very long on the floor and she was helped to a sitting position quite quickly although the sheet used to protect the dignity of female members wearing a skirt and who have fallen on the floor came out quite quickly after she fell to the floor.

Prior to this incident there was the usual invitation for prayer, after the speaker had finished speaking, where several members of the congregation went for prayer for deliverance or for healing. This church does not separate healing services from other services. (See observation of healing services in COGIC and URC in chapter 4 and above.) It is believed that messages (sermons) can be 'therapeutic' and healing takes place during the delivery of the sermon. Prayer is confirmation that healing has taken place for some people. The raised level of consciousness or the spiritual, psychological conditioning of the person during the service and the sermon prepares them for receiving healing or the completion of the healing process that started during the service.

There are similarities between the touch in the scenario with the COGIC minister and the touch by medical doctors and nurses to their patients in that both scenarios involve physical contact with the recipient. The doctor and the nurse rely on their professional training and their understanding of the human need to be touched whilst the minister relies on his connection with the Holy Spirit and his connection with the spirit of the recipient of prayer and healing. There are some apparent similarities demonstrated by the minister's minimum force when he placed his hand on the recipient's forehead as recorded in the extract from observation above.

This can be theorised by some to the complementary medicine theorists in the nursing journals as differences in the use of the energy field. Hallett (2004) describes this as the 'auric field' in the narratives of therapeutic touch he reports. Hallett suggests there are no direct physical side effects of this spiritual healing; however there is very often a feeling of wellness being experienced during and after treatment and many people experience warmth from the hands of the healer, yet on occasions a healer can convey a cool but not unpleasant effect. A gentle tingling sensation is often reported by patients (Hallett 2004). There are narratives of dramatic healing involving complete recovery or considerable improvement in a patient's conditions. Hallett, however, notes that on occasions, the symptoms of a particular condition become more pronounced for a short time in the aftermath of healing, due to the surfacing of tensions caused the complaint. Those he observed believed the aura of the healer touches the aura of the recipient and a cleansing that takes place in the 'auric' (or spiritual) field of the recipient. The cleansing could be the result of hearing a therapeutic message followed by being selected for prayer when the person was feeling alone and isolated.

The fact that the young lady at the COGIC convention reported above was selected for prayer and was given some information that appeared to be revealed by the spirit might be theorised as having made her receptive to the energies from the preacher. She had developed some trust in the preacher because he identified difficulties in her life that she had not told him. She may have developed trust in the spirit of the preacher because she was searching for someone to trust at that time when she was at a low and distressing time in her life. It is difficult to explain whether she believed wholeheartedly. However, there was no resistance when he took her by the hand and led her to the front of the audience. There was no force being used. He did not have to talk her into moving forward. She responded to his gentle request to move forward. She was probably reluctant to go forward during the first phase of prayer or in response to a general invitation. She needed some individual persuasion. She needed someone to recognize that she was going through a difficult time in her life. There may have been some facial features that the minister could see that no one else could see at that time.

This interaction has some similarities with Rogers' (1990) interpretation of transference and empathy where the client appears to be in control, but some transference of the broken spirit or emotional imbalance is transferred from the client (healed) and the counsellor (healer). The counsellor/healer uses empathy, therapeutic touch and prayer to heal the 'broken' spirit otherwise called low mood or clinical depression. Although psychotherapists do not frequently touch their clients, they use empathy in their therapy. A spiritual healer is expected to be use empathy as well as touch in the administration of healing (therapy). Unlike the scenarios in Hallett's (2004) study, I did not follow up my observation with the minister or with the recipient as this was not an experimental but an inductive study.

Conclusion: Let them all come!

In both churches, by using laying on of hands as a health promotion activity, healing is offered to everyone in the congregation including non-members. The approach is totally non-discriminatory. Both members and non-members engage in a health seeking behaviour when they volunteer for the healer to administer laying on of hands. In URC non—members are specially invited to the service on this day so that they can experience the power of Christian healing. Healing is theorised as available to people of whatever faith, colour, class or creed. Healing comes from a universal source of love and healers provide a channel for the healing energies to be passed to the patient. Healing occurs across the denominations and does not depend on the patient having any faith, religion or belief. It is given with love. This healing can be effected by contact with the patient or by means of absent, remote or distant healing. The healer allows himself/

Dr. Gwen Rose

herself as a channel for higher energy, which activates self—healing, power of the patient at relevant levels of many religions.

These two congregations do not promise cures and usually do not diagnose, but they have faith that there is some benefit to recipients as they practise the health seeking behaviour of laying on of hands. Spiritual healing is often used to support other forms of treatment that the patient may be receiving, from the General Practitioner or the hospital. Ministers/ healers of these two congregations will always encourage patients to follow or to continue treatment by their General Practitioners. In the churches, spiritual healing is a voluntary and free service as there are no medical fees to be paid through National insurance or any other scheme. There is no discrimination as healing using touch and anointing of oil is available to all and all are invited for healing whether there is a healing service or not.

Chapter Six

Music for Worship and Healing

Introduction

This chapter explores the therapeutic effects of music in worship and the practice of healing individuals which may differ according to their cultural and sociological background. It will draw on the study of religious music by Osterman (1998) which starts from her academic perspective as a university teacher of music, and also attempts a synthesis of sociology of religion, theology, and popular religious inspiration. The music used in each congregation that is examined and considered is music that is played for the purpose of worship and healing.

The use of music is more prominent within the COGIC Pentecostal church, where Music is one of the four main departments, the others being Missionary, Sunday school and Youth. The chapter will explore the feelings expressed by respondents about music and its therapeutic potential, using psychological narratives of the effect of music on the brain and cognition (Whitehouse 2005). Whitehouse argues that music has a direct effect on the brain and cognition and this discussion focuses on the role music in health promotion activity that is complementary to spiritual healing.

Music is mentioned twenty eight times in eight documents among the interview and fieldwork notes, and is indeed an integral part of each service observed. Music is also constituent of worship, even where there are no musical instruments, where there is singing for different purposes such as prayer, thanksgiving, celebration and worship. In the services observed in both churches music for worship is prominent as background music as well as music where some or all the congregation takes part. Evidence for the importance of music can be found in the orders of services for each church in section 3.

Contextualising the Origins of Worship Music

Both non-academic popular and serious academic theological accounts tend to give the legitimacy of antiquity to the healing effects of music, but sometimes, especially among evangelicals, there are warnings against "the devil's music". Muddiman's (2004) commentary on Paul's epistle to the Ephesians (and also on that to the Colossians) shows how the apostle emphasises the importance of speaking to each other in 'psalms, hymns and spiritual songs' as part of corporate worship.
Evangelical Christian theology often sees the use of music in worship as having been created in perfection with the angels but having then been made imperfect in part because of the angels, led by Satan, who became imperfect. Typical of this demonology are the writings of Dill (2003), which have since been cited on the internet. In Dill's attempt to identify 'the devil's music', he argues that the music that King of Tyre referred to in Ezekiel 28 is the same as Lucifer in Isaiah and that in both scriptures the angel is presented in a contradictory or sarcastic way as having high esteem as the son of the morning and at the same time the angel of destruction 'fallen from heaven and weakened the nations' creation of music reflecting satanic forces, so that music is not always of a positive healing or spiritual nature.

Doerkson (2004), the prolific worship music producer and performer, therefore suggests we consciously seek out music which is "A Journey into the Father's heart." He explains the inspiration for one of his song is the parable of the prodigal son and that his worship music is intended to bring the message of hope to those who are seeking a better life. The healing process may have started when the prodigal son decided to return to his father's house and continued when the father arranged a celebration with music as a welcome and forgiveness gesture. Musicians, hymnologists or song writers, he suggests, are inspired by a spiritual force that represents the heart of God. Although such inspiration is not something that can be empirically researched the music observed in both churches could be viewed in the way Doerkson suggests. Musicians were dedicated and committed to the worship music that they played. In the services observed in both churches music for worship is prominent as background music as well as a fore-grounded performance in which some or all the congregation takes part.

Pullar (1988) in her Penguin guide to spiritual healing for lay people, which attempts to take an objective stance, gives an account of how singing (background music) contributes to the healing process, as in the following instance: *'The healer stirred round in the patient's mouth and lifted the offending tooth as though it was lying there loose and waiting to be removed. Next he massaged the swollen glands in the patient's throat and made him sit back with his mouth wide open while he began to sing to him softly'.* Stacy et al (2002), as health educators, uphold the claim that singing specifically has health-giving properties. The founder of the Healing Music Organisation in California, Amitra Cottrell (2005) claims she was healed from cancer through singing to herself, and argues that music has played a significant role in healing since the beginning of recorded history. Famous historic figures such as Plato and Pythagoras, are mentioned, with their appreciation of Apollo, the god of both medicine and music, appealing to the oft-cited, but never-referenced 'famous quote' from Plato that "Music is a moral law. It gives soul to the Universe, wings to the mind, flight to the imagination, a charm to sadness and life to everything. It is the essence of order that leads to all that is good and beautiful, of which it is beautiful, but nevertheless passion in an eternal form"[3]. Priestly (1975) in her psychoanalytic approach concurs that studying the cathartic and hypnotic uses of music through history and in all cultures indicates that music must have been used therapeutically.

Littlewood et al (2000), in comparing psychoanalysis with shamanic healing, cite Levi-Strauss's (1993) discussion of the use of songs amongst other symbols that are used to help women with a difficult childbirth. The suggestion is that the physical effects of music may complement the

---

[3] The author cannot find any passage resembling this anywhere in the complete English translations of Plato on the internet. It would be interesting to know who actually composed these words, and who first attributed the sentiment to Plato, but it is not necessary to support the argument of this thesis.

symbolic effects of ritual, which may perhaps parallel the way healers can suggest that physical and spiritual interventions are complementary.

Osterman (1998) asserts 'The body is the temple of God therefore music in the body should be music in the temple." In a study in which she is frank about her personal religious inspiration, she attempts a critical scholarly and scientific approach, providing a detailed account of the biological, social and spiritual aspects of worship music. She maintains that 'music is organized sound, governed by time and space, creates and influence feelings, ideas, emotions, moods and behaviour. Sound is an external stimulus that activates the senses through vibrations. These vibrations produce mental images, memories and physical responses' (Osterman 1998:94). She considers two categories of music; liturgical or functional worship music and non-liturgical music based on religious themes but not necessarily intended for worship.

Music is an essential part of church worship and spiritual healing as health seeking behaviour, and is of course part of the link between specific worship/ritual activities and everyday life. As Moodley and West (2005:5) say in their book on integrating traditional healing practices with counselling and psychotherapy, 'In some cultures music is used to ward off evil spirits'. Music is used to bring calm and peace, to worship, to dispel evil and bring us closer to God as is shown in the work of Roseman (1991), Kirkpatrick (1996) and others discussed Chapter 2. Hutson (2000) postulates that although not explicitly a healing ritual, the rave in Western youth subculture has been claimed as a form of healing, comparable both with shamanic healing and with spiritual experiences.

There is, in fact, an interchange between music used for religious purposes and music used for other purposes. This can sometimes be controversial when secular or "profane" music is appropriated for religious purposes or indeed the other way round. Beckford (2006) explores the 'dialogue' between African-Caribbean dance hall and church hall, in his examination of the origins of black majority Pentecostal church music, and shows how religious music can be ambiguous about its use of secular techniques, even as secular music borrows gospel themes.

Osterman (1998) and Etherington (2003) both give accounts of music or singing meetings among Black slaves where music was popular particularly for those who could not read or write. Such music created important focal points of social interaction. Prior to the emancipation of the slaves, such activities were called 'tea meetings.' Prayer meetings in COGIC appears to have similar functions.

Extract from observation
First song 332 from the Redemption Songs: I need no other argument—
4th verse: My great physician heals
Second song: 567
All songs were prayerful with a slow tempo. There is no music in the prayer meeting and the fasting services. The group members rely on their knowledge of the song therefore at least two people must know the song and have the confidence to sing and let the others follow their lead.

MacRobert (1988) describes how the extensive use of instrumental music, drumming, singing and dancing are associated with rituals as a religious expression of receiving the Spirit in many African countries as well as the New World. Drumming, singing and dancing passed into the Negro Spiritual for the slaves in the West Indies and America, representing a theological, political, social, historical and cultural inheritance, although Europeans made every effort to reduce it to the conventional musical notation which characterised western hymnody and secular music. Nonetheless, the embodiment of biblical themes in the Negro Spiritual enabled Black people to transcend enslavement and look to God for liberation and freedom from oppression.

For Pentecostals, music, singing and shouting open up the worshipper to the power of the divine. Beckford's (2006) exposition of the politics of sound confirm that sound is never merely a noise but is the foundation of different cultures and can only be decoded according to the specific cultural values and interpretation. He uses the sound of Jamaican dancehall music in his illustration of the inter-related and inter-dependent power of sound where Christians were resistant to dancehall sound, but nonetheless could not be immune to the meanings of music derived from their own cultures. This arguably can be applied to all cultures, especially if music is viewed as part of people and their culture.

Beckford's approach has some similarities with biblical scholars' exposition of the cultural origins of music mentioned in the New Testament. Early Christian music had its own origin in cultural traditions. In Ephesians, Paul implores the believers at Ephesus to 'speak to each other in psalms, hymns and spiritual songs, singing and chanting in your hearts.' Muddiman's (2004) exposition of Ephesians asserts that hymns and spiritual songs were synonymous with psalms. These were already used in Jewish worship and were adapted for Christian worship. In their commentaries, Constable (2008) and Guthrie (2003) both suggest that spiritual songs put God in control and when God controls us we are joyful. With spiritual songs and joy comes healing.

Mood Enhancing Medical Treatment: the Effects of Opioids

Community relationships elicit endogenous opioid mechanisms (Frecska 1989), with effects on consciousness and health, including immune-system responses. Healing rituals use emotionally charged cultural symbols that have been cross-conditioned with physiological and emotional responses, the endocrine system, and the immune system, linking the psychic/mythological and somatic spheres (Frecska 1989). Brain opioid systems provide neuro-chemical mediation of social bonding. Frecska suggested that shamanic healing practices utilize complex forms of opioid-mediated attachment to promote psychobiological synchrony within the group, reinforcing identification and the internalization of social relations.

Some doctors prescribe an exercise with music programmes arguing that this is more effective than medication for the depressed patient such as flouxetine hydrochloride (prozac)[4] which takes two weeks for the patient

---

[4] Prozac is classified as an antidepressant with a selective inhibitor of serotonin re-uptake (BMA/BPS2009). It also has mood enhancing properties. It has no affinity to other receptors and is absorbed well after oral administration. Peak plasma concentration is reached in 6-8 hours and it is strongly bound to plasma protein. Steady state plasma concentration is achieved after ingesting the drug for several weeks as prescribed. It is extensively metabolised in the

to experience any significant reduction of their depression. Lynch (2004) and Linnett (2005) both reject the traditional medical approach to depression and view it as an emotional, spiritual and existential crisis. It being a spiritual crisis (a cry for spiritual help), they suggest that spiritual intervention can be of some benefit to the person suffering from depression or one with a depressive illness. However they stress that music and spiritual intervention should not replace medical intervention and drugs where necessary.

Much of this literature is summed up by Whitehouse and Macauley (2005), who postulate four distinct ways in which our brain responds to music as cognitive, affective, personal and transpersonal. In other words we respond to music by feeling the music with our emotions (cognitive, affective), by noticing the effect on our heart rate and breathing (physical) and feeling the connection with God (transpersonal) though music. The senses are activated by a stimulus in the sense organs of the skin, ears, eyes, mouth and nose and a receptor in the brain. This in turn is recorded in the memory and classified before a response is produced by the person. The ear is the most sensitive organ and is activated before birth. It has been recorded that the unborn child responds to noises around the mother and when music is played near to the surface of the pregnant woman's abdomen, the foetus can be seen on ultrasound or scan to make different movements from when there is absolute quiet. A young child who is familiar with certain noises will sleep during such noises. If the noise becomes unfamiliar the person's sleep will be disturbed.

Hanser (1990) found that music can provide a positive stimulus for depressed older adults and Lai (1999) observed that music elicits tranquil mood states in depressed women. A spiritual healer during the healing ritual utilizes the capacity of music on innate brain modules associated with call and vocalization systems manifested in singing and chanting (Wallin, Merker, and Brown 1999; Molino 2000). These expressive systems based in rhythm and affective dynamics communicate emotional states, and

---

liver to nor-fluxotene and a number of identified metabolites, which are excreted in the urine (MIMS Nurses 2007, BMA/BPS 2009).

motivate others' responses, enhancing group cohesion, synchronization, and cooperation (Geissrnann 1999).

Music appears to have an important and pivotal role in the healing processes of many cultures and in particular folk medicine and, in more recent times, relaxation therapies such as massage and aromatherapies. Wallin, et al (2000) and Molino (2000,) found that music has a positive effect on listeners' self-reported depression, fatigue and overall mood. They also observed its definite effects in the reduction of anxiety among people with chronic obstructive pulmonary disease. Molino (2000) drawing on Donald (1991) suggested that the practices of music, dancing, and ritual imitation establish group coordination through rhythmo-affective semantics that express fundamental emotions. The feeling of togetherness that communal music indicates that feeling part of a system such as a style of music has healing effects on what could be homeostatic imbalance in illness and dis-ease. The effect of music in the release of opioids is responsible for carrying out the biological effects of music. The release of natural opioids and serotonin stimulates the immunological system and produces a sense of euphoria, certainty, and belongingness.

A wide range of ritual healing activities induces the production and release of endogenous opioids which have similar mood enhancing properties as some antidepressants such as Prozac (Linnett 2005). Ritual music for healing produces the release of endogenous opioids through exhaustive rhythmic movement (e.g., dancing and clapping); temperature extremes (cold or sweat lodges); austerities (water and food deprivation, flagellation, self-inflicted wounds); emotional manipulations (fear and positive expectations); and night time activities, when endogenous opioids are naturally highest (Prince 1982, Winkelman 1998 and 2000). Valle and Raymond (1989) and Prince (1982) hypothesized that endogenous opioids enhance coping skills, maintenance of bodily homeostasis, pain reduction, stress tolerance, environmental adaptation, and group psychobiological synchronization.

Physiological Effects of Music

According to Osterman (1998), music can influence the nervous system without affecting the brain. Sound waves and sympathetic vibrations on the ear drums are transformed to chemical and nerve impulses which register different sounds that we hear. They give shock in rhythmical sequence to muscles which cause them to contract and set our arms, legs and feet in motion. These activities elicit physical responses such as an increase of sexual stimulus, or hunger or thirst; or they may have a calming or healing result. Osterman cites Louis R. Torres, the distinguished Seventh Day Adventist seminary teacher, and former bass guitarist of Bill Haley and the Comets as asserting 'The roots of the auditory nerves are more widely distributed and have more extensive connections than those of any other nerve in the body most of our body functions are affected by the pulsations and harmonic effects of musical tones' (Torres and Torres 1997:18). However the spoken word must pass through the master brain to be interpreted and screened for musical content: therefore music with words may not have the same effect on the autonomic nervous system.

Waugh (2006) describes the neurones in the autonomic nervous system as operating like electrical impulses. These act as neuro-chemical transmitters affecting specific body parts and in turn affect the muscles, bladder, circulation, sex organs, gall bladder and all the body organs such as the skin, kidneys stomach and spleen. The Aetherius Society 'Bishop', Richard Lawrence (2001) uses these physiological facts to claim fear, hate and anger are negative emotions that weaken the thymus gland. More credibly, Diamond (1998) discusses how the skin, which is the largest organ in the body, is affected by fear and therefore when the person is exposed to music which invokes positive or negative emotion the whole body is likely to be affected. Osterman (1998) and Diamond (1998) both argue that music as an aspect of our physical environment has an effect upon our health and wellbeing and the body is able to discriminate between beneficial and detrimental sounds. This is probably true in the same way that the body can benefit from medicine but not other ingested material that is detrimental. People can become so involved in a particular type of music (especially those that depress the nervous system) without consciously realising that they are causing damage and not healing. The thymus gland is more active in young people than in the adults. Therefore the process of selecting music that is long lasting is more intense in a young person. This may explain why some music is regarded as 'music of the decade (era)' as the music is remembered by a generation of people who were between the ages of 15-25 years.

The state of animation exhibited by people worshipping in Pentecostal churches, such as COGIC, indicates the possibility of an altered state of consciousness (ASC). There are attendees who have a regular pattern of behaviour which is specifically reserved for church services. During singing, clapping, shouting, and chanting "praise the Lord" stimulated by gospel music, they may engage in speaking in tongues (glossolalia) falling to the floor (being slain in the spirit) and experience limb and muscle tremor. This could be viewed as a cleansing process or the casting out of demonic spirits as described in section3. Rayburn and Richmond (2002) suggest altered states of consciousness are elicited when the nervous system responds to injury or fatigue or excitement. Prior to this altered state of consciousness, information is transmitted from the behavioural part of the brain into the rest of the body. The message and the response are personally and culturally interpreted. The altered state of consciousness in worship can result in a sense of connectedness, oneness and personal integration with a higher force.

Sound can have physical effects on the matter in our body in the same way that it may sometimes break glass. Sound is transmitted to the brain through the auditory nerve which may reach the autonomic nervous system. Graham (1999) suggests that the rhythmic auditory stimuli of drumming practised by Native American or Eastern Buddhist mantra chanting may induce an altered mental and physical state.

Ward (1989) suggests the altered state of consciousness is different from person to person in the same way that the 'normal' state of conscious is different for each person. The altered state of consciousness could be described as a hypnotic trance, sleep, rapid eye movement (dream state) daydreaming meditation where people do not remember the events occurring during the time they were experiencing muscle tremor or other evidence of an altered state of consciousness. "ASC" can be induced through different methods other than music and chanting such as opiods, anti-depressants, or hallucinogens breathing exercises, deprivations associated with fasting, self sacrifice, and isolation.

ASC experiences can be elicited naturally because of the nervous system responses to injury, extreme fatigue, near starvation, or ingestion of hallucinogens or because of a wide variety of deliberate procedures such as drumming, chanting, music, fasting, sensory deprivation, or deliberate sleep (Winkelman 1998). Winkelman (2000) describes the physiology of ASCs in some detail. They activate the limbic system producing a parasympathetic dominant state of deep relaxation and internal focus of attention. ASCs stimulate the serotonergic nervous system exemplified in the action of meditation and psycho-integrators (hallucinogens) upon the brain. This in turn can activate the autonomic nervous system resulting in a parasympathetic dominant state of relaxation of the serotonin receptors, with their highest nerve concentrations in the lower brain, the limbic system hippocampus and amygdala, and the frontal cortex's visual and auditory areas which act as a modulatory system across levels of the brain. Important effects of serotonin are the integration of emotional and motivational processes and the synthesis of information across the functional levels of the brain. The overall effect of ASC is to integrate information from the whole organism. This specifically involves transmitting information from the emotional and behavioural preverbal brain structures into the personal and cultural systems mediated by language and the frontal cortex. Theologians (Rottschaefer 1999, Rayburn and Richmond 2002) looking at the physiology of ASCs have suggested these biological conditions provide a basis for experiences of enlightenment, a sense of connection and oneness, and personal integration

Music as Therapy

Music as a therapy is described by Priestly (1975) and Harrison (2004) as including three factors: the client, the music and the therapist. Where there are only two, the client and the music, the experience may be therapeutic but not therapy as in the sense of someone administering therapy (taking care of another person or persons). Consequently, the human relationship is important in any aspect of therapy as that relationship is the therapy. There may be other contributory factors such as prayer, oils, or touch which can be viewed as tools, aids or adjuncts to the therapy. The success or failure of the therapy is dependent on the success of the human and spiritual relationships that are applied. In using music to assist the therapy and the therapist in spiritual healing, the experience for both therapist and client can be enriching or destructive. The therapists who use music to assist in their work needs to use music that is soothing and within the comfort zone of the client. As it is the therapist who usually chooses the music, the choice has to be also within the comfort zone of the therapist. In other words the music cannot be irritating, depressing or reflect negative emotions in the therapist. The therapist should aim to promote calm and positive emotions in the client. If the therapist is comfortable, it is more likely that the client will be comfortable with the selected music.

There are CDs of recorded music for healing to accompany various healing treatments and music to accompany what is seen as the revival of ancient healing methods that are becoming accepted in today's climate of increased stress from busy lifestyles where people crave and need more time for peace and tranquillity. There is music to promote tranquillity, harmonious living, inner peace and better concentration as well as better sleep and relaxation. Appropriate recorded music is sometimes used for healing services in the URC when the organist or pianist is unavailable.

Music therapy works for clients in different ways, iIn the same way as each individual responds to a particular type of medicine or foods in a different way. Some of the ways that music works for clients are listed by Priestley (1975): assisting the client with communication difficulties to improve their communication; changing the environment so that the focus is not on the illness and the client can enjoy an environment that transcends his present world; helping the client who is out of touch with reality to get back in touch with reality. In some cases the client cannot say what or how music works; he just knows that it works. Priestley further explains that it is only in the past decade that music has been officially accepted in this country as an ancillary medical service. He argues that music therapy harmoniously integrates the ego, super-ego and id of Freud's conceptual model of the psyche. Priestley and the pop psychologist Campbell (1998) argue that as music is a part of our existence, just being alive and aware as a human being promotes inner music. 'Melody exists in the soul of man. The soul is indeed the harp upon which the musician plays. The whole body of man is a musical instrument on which Ego resounds and the soul produces melody, therefore melody lies within man himself' (Priestley 1975:200). Priestley (1975:18) pre-empted Beckford's (2006) view of music and drums in the statement "Group drumming experiences can bring players in touch with deep levels of the collective unconscious as can folk dance music from the ethnic group."

In Christian churches worship with and through music is endemic as part of the human spirit. Music creates a natural and enriched environment and makes it easier for the healer to operate. When the body is relaxed, festering negative thoughts are brought to the surface. The empty space is replaced by good thoughts which have healing effects. The healer or therapist can intuitively sense harmony or conflict with the client. It is difficult to analyze the music that is used in the Pentecostal church as there are so many different instruments used. However it is clear that the combination sounds produces the desired effect on the people from their own cultural perspective. Music during focused prayer is slower than music during a testimony service.

The environment for spiritual healing which promotes health seeking and health enhancing behaviour differs between the two churches as was noted in chapter 4 and this extends to their musical cultures. In COGIC, the musical instruments of drums, organ, guitar, trumpet and an additional keyboard are situated to the right of the rostrum and the choir is situated to the left. The praise and worship team sit stand on the right in front of the musical instruments. The instruments used in the URC are mainly organ, the piano and occasionally the guitar. The organ is situated towards the back on the right and there is also a piano at the front on the right side. The choir usually sits to the back of the church near the organist.

COGIC services commonly resound with spirited expressions of emotion and powerfully hypnotic music employing repetitive chanted phrases. These melodies are seen as expressing the emotions of the soul of the people of African descent. According to Harvey (2005) ordinary gospel hymns are transformed to a song that is typically African in its accompaniment with clapping hands, feet tapping and singing style.

The literature on the therapeutic effects of the specific music that is played in either church is limited, although the respondents, particularly the organist in the URC, gave clear indications of their belief in the therapeutic effect of music. Worship music is believed to make a contribution to the healing process and the healing process in the services is enhanced through worship music. Rice and Huffstattler (2001) sum up music as being an organic part of daily life. They suggest worship music disappeared and reappeared over time in the early and modern Christian church.

The Pentecostal style of worship music is one where there is a 'band' or group of different instruments that accompanies the praise and worship music. Although there is now more acceptance of having a band of musicians in the non-Pentecostal churches the concept of praise and worship teams has not yet arrived on a large scale in many non-Pentecostal churches. The URC congregation in the study has not adopted this style of worship.

The extracts from fieldwork notes below illustrate the process of worship music that can affect healing in COGIC.

'The first song was slow and sung prayerfully. The hymns were led by the Praise and Worship team. This team consist of three female singers, one male singer and the instrumentalists (organist, drummer and guitarist). They are younger members and do not have a uniform unless they are singing with the choir. They do not sit in a separate section like the choir. The choir which is different from the Praise and Worship team consists of primarily older female members (12 female and three male) and also includes members of the team. They sit to the left of the congregation on the first level of the rostrum. They dress uniformly in black and white. Some members of the team write songs for the group and also select hymns for the choir.

Not all the members of the singing group were present at the start of the service. Like everyone else they joined the group and the service later than the official starting time. There were 18 people present when the service started at 10.35 am. The minister and an elder emerged from the vestry following the preparation for service. As they entered the church, the organist played a musical rendition and the congregation was silent (some members prayed silently during this time).

The atmosphere at the COGIC convention rally was not very different to the ordinary congregational services observed. There, too, prayer for healing, accompanied by a petition that the Holy Spirit might enter the worshippers, was an intrinsic part of the service and background music was very prominent.

The extract below from an observation of a healing service illustrates the standard process at the beginning of all URC services. The variation in a healing service comes at the end of the service when church attendees are invited to come to the front of the church for healing through prayer and the laying of hands.

The minister enters from the vestry as the organist plays a musical rendition. He is dressed in black clerical attire. The service starts promptly on time. He welcomes the congregation and introduces the healing service.

The minister reads psalms 108:1-6 from the New International Version of the bible (the pew bible) together with the congregation as a call to worship. Part of the regular order of the service is the call to worship (Jones 2002).

The music seen as therapeutic in the URC draws on a different cultural tradition, which emphasizes a very different style of music. There is a wide body of "complementary" (Campbell 1998) and "new age" (Cottrell 2005) thought which has exaggerated and capitalised commercially on the tentative scientific work of Tomatis (1991) and Rauscher, et al (1993). This provides a secular version of narrative about the practice, therapeutic, cathartic and hypnotic uses of music through history and in most cultures discussed by Priestly (1975). Within this tradition Campbell (1998) has actually called the alleged therapeutic input "The Mozart effect".

In COGIC the singing is accompanied by moving of the body when standing, and shaking of the head when sitting. There are also prayerful songs with a slower instrumental accompaniment contrasting with more celebratory music that has a faster tempo. The music in the URC also reflects the different culture of its people. The act of worship through music is no less powerful or real to either congregation. However, to a person who has been culturally conditioned to worship with quiet music a more varied kind of music may not be acceptable.

Some of the older Pentecostals members believe that music that is not played in church is 'devil worship music'. They see a strong contrast between music that is used for good and music that is used for evil. Worshipping through music, however, has the potential to lift the emotions and the spirit and consequently stimulate the immune system to aid the healing process.

When there were no actual musical instruments, the participants used their voices in singing hymns which produced musical sounds. This is illustrated in the observation of the fasting and prayer meeting in COGIC (extract below).

First hymn 332 from the Redemption Songs: I need no other argument—
4th verse: My great physician heals . . . .
Second song: 567
All hymns were prayerful with a slow tempo. There is no instrumental music in the prayer meeting and the fasting services. The group members rely on their knowledge of the song therefore at least two people must know the song and have the confidence to sing and let the others follow their lead.

Respondent 5, the organist in the URC often used her own initiatives when playing music at the beginning and at the end of the services as a preparation or close to worship and healing services. She experienced music as therapy but described it in a more down-to-earth way than the genteel approaches in Priestley's (1975) exposition of music therapy. For her, the relationship with other people, with music as a catalyst, is the therapy. Below, she describes how music, fellowship, worship and friendliness of the church attendees made her feel useful when she was feeling low and despondent. She also described how redundant she felt when she was not allowed to play music in one church and how her faith was restored when she was asked to play music in her current church where she took membership. She did not have much academic understanding of music and healing but she certainly understood the effect of music on the congregation and on herself during the services whether or not she was playing personally. Priestley (1975) and Hanser (2005a, 2005b) explain how the effects of music on the person in a more academic and detailed way, as the acting out of emotions with some control through a guilt-free medium of non-verbal sound. Respondent 5 could act out her guilt through her music and the hymns which are sung during worship and healing services.

Respondent 5 (URC): *'I was looking after my mother and my husband who by this time had a mental problem. He was diagnosed with Alzheimer's disease. I could not give all my devotion to him as he had done when I was ill.(I felt guilty) I should not have done but I felt that I did not have enough energy to support him the way he had supported me when I was ill. Then my mum died the same year I had my heart operation. So I felt that I had reached rock bottom again.'*

This respondent experienced grief and loss through her husband's illness, her mother's death and her own illness. The church that she attended at the time compounded this loss by preventing her from playing music possibly on the premise that they were helping her by relieving her of her duties (see below). By being relieved of her duties she was made to feel redundant, useless. Although she was probably feeling helpless as a result of not being able change the course of the illnesses in her family, removing her from music was like removing a very important aspect of her treatment (a built in therapy that had become a necessary component that affected the outcome of treatment for all the tragedies in her life in one year).

The extract below illustrates the effect on the church attendee when her primary role was taken from her when other areas of her life were not going well. She experienced healing through her contribution of playing music in the church and healing services. She confirms Cottrell's (2005) view that music stirs emotional feelings and helps to deal with sadness, grief, anger and other feelings.

Respondent 5 URC: *'I was involved with the music and this was taken away from me. Consequently as a result of this and other things I did not feel supported by the church during a very difficult time in my life. I left the church as a result of this'*

This respondent's approach to worship music provided continuous healing for her. She was bereft when she could not play music that was an integral part of her life in church. When she was allowed to play in a different church, the healing process started for different reasons. While simply being allowed to feel useful again was a healing factor, it is possible music in itself contributed to the healing of the pain and hurt in her life.

What emerged from this respondent is that her healing is an integral part of church service and church life. The music, the fellowship, the worship, friendliness, and being made to feel helpful when one is feeling helpless and despondent all go together.

Interviewer: When you are playing music do you perceive the type of music that is needed for a particular moment in a healing service?
Respondent 5 URC: 'I could not stand up and preach a sermon but I could preach a sermon through a song.
Interviewer: So, it sounds like the change in itself was like a healing?
Respondent: Yes, the fact that I was not in the environment where I was resentful got rid of that feeling of resentfulness. I feel very much at home here. In the other church I was involved in the music and that was taken away for me. I did not feel that I had any purpose to go there, to sing to play the piano. I still meet up with the people from the church
But I don't get asked to join in with anything as I used to do.
Interviewer: I am interested in the music. Can you tell me more about that I can see that you are really interested in music? Do you think music in itself contributes to healing.
Respondent: I used to play for the Sunday school so I have played church music all my life.

The passage cited from Respondent 10 (COGIC) a member of the Praise and Worship team—in chapter 2 section 3 above also illustrates and concurs with Respondent 5 from URC that those who have a musical or singing role in the church and are then excluded from participating in worship music, can become depressed and feel useless. When Respondent 5 from URC was re-instated to play music and sing, her depression seem to be healed. When respondent 10 from COGIG was healed and returned to singing she felt better about herself and her belief in divine healing. The role of music for them appears to be an important part of their existence. They believe that where they cannot preach or pray they make a valuable contribution to worship and healing through music.

Conclusion

The chapter has discussed the importance of music in worship which surrounds spiritual healing and as a therapeutic tool in itself. The interrogation of the sociological, clinical, theological and popular religious discourses shows that they all present narratives that music can get people 'in the mood' to be receptive and accept healing in different environments and for different conditions. Some of these conditions are anxiety, depression and other physical illnesses. To say this is not to confirm the bolder claims about therapeutic outcomes for any particular kind of music because, as for prayer, there are many obstacles to controlled experiments or observation of the actual effect of music on individuals during worship and healing services. Music was a common factor in all the worship and healing services observed. When there were no actual musical instruments, the participants used their voices in singing hymns which produced musical sounds. Although not tested in rigorously controlled double-blind procedures, there may be some evidence that music and dance contribute to the release of endogenous opioids which have mood enhancing properties and therefore could be a contributory factor in the healing process.

Chapter Seven

Conclusion

Introduction

This thesis has focussed on the limitations of the discussion of spiritual healing in health and health promotion models which are promoted and practised by medical and health professionals. The vision of the researcher was intended to highlight the gap and bring to the attention of the statutory authorities and church ministers the need to recognise the importance of spiritual healing as a health promotion activity amongst church attenders. She chose to investigate one black majority and one white majority congregation and compare and contrast their practice in administering and receiving spiritual healing. The following sections outline the contents of the chapters of the thesis and the result of the investigation.

The Vision

The first chapter provided a summary of the ethnographic approach taken in this research where the researcher starts and finishes the process as part of the subject and the environment being investigated. This study was prompted by the opportunity of drawing together my health professional and life experiences as well as researching the people who form a large part of my life. I, like them, brought experience and ideas, like Lévi-Strauss's (1966) *bricoleur*, from anywhere that seemed to work. The thesis has itself taken a *bricolage* approach which includes several disciplines where literature and the arts are used to construct models and narratives of healing from a diverse range of sources. This diversity includes literature on healing from many levels, both academic and popular, concerning medicine, nursing, theology, sociology and anthropology.

During my professional and Christian life, teaching health promotion to nurses and other allied health professionals, and as a member of a Pentecostal church, the separation of spiritual healing from other health practices was identified. It was not appropriately addressed in the classroom, or the church where it appeared to be in isolation from any statutory health input. Clients did not and still do not feel that they could mention their beliefs to their health professionals and the latter are not allowed to mention spiritual healing. This was particularly alienating where the clients were black and the health professionals white. It is argued that the black and ethnic minority population feel marginalised in the way they receive healthcare in the same way they feel marginalised in the workplace.

Awareness of the lack of research and the existence of a neglected oral tradition within the Pentecostal black majority churches was also a motivating factor. I wanted to make a contribution to knowledge by adding some insight and possibly literature on the subject of the spiritual healing which is regularly practised in church services but not addressed in the classroom of health professionals or health promotion authors. Beyond the research, I wished personally to give some input to endeavours to bridge the gap between health professionals and church attenders, especially those from black majority churches.

The Process

The literature review reported in chapter 2 set the parameters for the investigation and identified the gaps in the material which warrant the methodology descrsibed in Chapter 3. Although all of these areas have been addressed in the relevant literature, they needed fleshing out and bringing together to provide a context for understanding how members of these churches integrate their various health-seeking behaviours.

- the existing oral tradition of the Pentecostal church. Members learn through practice and under the supervision of older members and ministers compared with the more book-centred approach of mainstream Protestantism.

- the 'realised', 'last days' eschatology of the Pentecostal belief system where people practise their faith without questioning that promises of healing can be fulfilled, and the aspirational eschatology of mainstream Protestantism which leads to different expectations of spiritual healing.
- the ways in which health seeking behaviour through spiritual healing is pursued at the same time as the seeking of medical advice.
- the way church attenders may feel diffident about discussing their belief in prayer with their doctor or other health professionals

As Hammersley (1993) infers may happen, as the researcher I consistently felt like an outsider. At no time has the sense of being a stranger been lost and therefore I have had to maintain a critical analytic perspective. As a counsellor I expected to have times when I felt empathetic and at 'ease' with the subjects (the respondents and the research environments) but these times were very short and very few. There are, however, two distinct difficult aspects, one writing as a critical observer and the other adjusting to the periodic and short times when I felt 'at home.' The research processes has also involved a spiritual journey which is not easily described because this journey has been sporadic with times when an understanding of the world around me has been elusive.

My inquisitive nature as a child has continued and will continue throughout all aspects of my life. Giving my research an ethnographic label and placing it in an academic setting has not altered my life's purpose and journey; it has been enhanced with an improved body of knowledge. I can see much of Hammersley's (1993) and Brewer's (2000) exposition of the principles and practice of ethnography reflected in my research experience. Although the environment was familiar, the role of ethnographic researcher was unfamiliar and required re-socialisation into the practices and values of the group (c.f. Brewer 2000). Prior to this understanding, these principles were unsubstantiated readings and feelings. Now I can relate Hammersley's and Brewer's writings to my research journey and life experiences.

After seven years, of concentrated thought about matters of health promotion and their desirable relatedness to spiritual healing, I have only begun to scratch the surface. There is a desperate need for further research in the areas that have been highlighted such as prayer, laying of hands, music and the cultural background and theology, in particular of black majority Pentecostal churches.

The initial aim of the study: 'to explore the perceptions of church attenders in the two churches' has been achieved within the remit of the research methodology. It is difficult to measure 'perception' without a complex psychological tool designed for this purpose. An ethnographic approach is not a research design to gain access to the private aspect of these people's lives, but rather to their collective understandings. The study was not designed to study psychological phenomena but to apply a sociological, theological and anthropological approach. The experience of this study could provide a springboard to a scientific psychological study using appropriately designed tools.

The Outcome: Similarities and Differences

There are similarities and differences between COGIC, a black majority church, and the mainstream, white majority URC in their approaches to the administration and delivery of spiritual healing.

Section two provides a comparison of the two churches in terms of their history, doctrine and belief in spiritual healing. To some extent they conformed to the images presented in the literature that the connection between physical healing and spiritual healing is a constant feature of Pentecostalism (Tugwell et al 1976), whereas, as Rice and Huffstatler (2001) comment, spiritual healing is a neglected form of pastoral care in the mainstream Protestant churches. Although Pentecostal churches haves Protestant origins, their approach to healing is different and is viewed as a part of grace and salvation which every believer has the right to claim.

Both Tugwell et al (1976) and Rice and Huffstatler (2001) point out that consciousness of the connection between sickness and sin in the scriptures has survived in the Reformed tradition as well as in Pentecostalism. Rice and Huffstatler (2001) interestingly observe that the healing ministry almost disappeared from the mainstream church (apart perhaps from the rite of the last sacrament (*viaticum*) administered to the dying) but has in the last few decades returned to many older Christian churches. This was perhaps prompted by the fact that at the same time as the disappearance of the healing ministry in the mainstream Protestant churches, the healing ministry in the Pentecostal churches had gathered momentum.

The different approach to healing between COGIC and URC suggests that cultural differences in worship style are as important as differences in doctrine. With reference to spiritual healing, these varying practices may in part derive from the fact that many URC members have the capacity to articulate their thoughts to a nuanced understanding of the relationship between spiritual and physical health. In COGIC, as the majority of the church attenders are not able (or choose not to) develop their thoughts on explaining miraculous healing; they are more ready to accept the statement 'it was a miracle' without any further explanation.

The Pentecostals believe that healing is inherent in salvation and both are possible in an instant or over a period of time, whereas, an URC member are more likely to believe that healing takes place over a period of time and is less likely to be instantaneous. Although the minister is expected to sanction healing activities, the importance of a healing ministry remains a matter of individual perception and choice. The need to make healing a part of worship services a priority, or appointing spiritual healers can be sidelined if the resident minister attaches too little attention to such matters.

In section two, consideration was given to the role of the minister, organisational culture and the concept of power and control in church governance and spiritual healing at different levels; local, national and international levels in both churches were all explored. The finding of an overt link between healing and salvation in COGIC, the Pentecostal church, that is different to the URC, illustrates the different cultures and theologies of the observed congregations.

COGIC ministers 'allow' the Holy Spirit to guide the church services with reference to the length of service which they often extend over a longer period of time. This however may be a result of the cultural background of the people who want to take time without limitation to worship God. This non-limitation of time may also be a contributing factor to their claim for healing. The order of the service may also change as a result of 'the direction of the Holy Spirit'. This maybe because the minister cannot explain a reason for the change and the worship style of visitation of the Holy Spirit, as on the day of Pentecost and later in the Azusa Street revival which legitimate their liturgical norms.

Chapter 2 examined suffering as an outcome of imbalance in homeostasis and one of the causal factors for people to seek spiritual healing. When exploring suffering it is found that it is inextricably linked with faith and healing, now or in the afterlife for those who believe in an afterlife. The 'Apostles' Creed', written when the early Christians suffered much persecution and were forced to renounce their faith under anti-Christian laws, acknowledges the suffering of Christ, the forgiveness of sin (and suffering) and life everlasting. The Nicene Creed is a revised version of the Apostles' Creed and was adopted in the time of Constantine when Christianity became the official religion of the Roman Empire (Young 1993). Both churches use creeds as the foundation of their Christian doctrine and as a means of solemnising membership of the church. The chapter discusses the culture-bound facets of suffering and the different perceptions of suffering by the respondents. There is an indication that spiritual healing can move people psychologically from the suffering caused by generations of abuse or addiction such as alcohol through acknowledgement and forgiveness.

Chapters, 4, 5 and 6 focuses on the outcomes of the processes of prayer, music and laying of hands as health promotion activities and considers how these relate to the illness action models reviewed by Kasl and Kolb (1996) and the definitions of health and health behaviour models by Dingwall (1976).

During the healing services when prayer, music and the laying of hands are used to administer healing, people may seem to enter an altered state of consciousness when they are one with God and the Universe. This experience may be present only momentarily, although the person may not recognise the change until minutes, hours or days later.

The optimum health and absence of disease as described by Seedhouse (1992), Blaxter (1995), Dubois (1995) and Janzen (1992) cannot be sustained for any period of time. This may explain why health seeking-behaviours of consultation with doctors, other health professionals and spiritual healers have to be repeated to effect continuous healing throughout life until what may be regarded as the ultimate healing of death.

Models of health-seeking behaviour now present a broader view of human behaviour than Parsons' (1975) model of illness behaviour and the sick role. Working women are often reluctant to adopt the sick role as they find it difficult to withdraw from their social roles of mothering and domestic tasks. Many church attenders, probably because they are mostly women, are also reluctant to adopt the sick role if it involves withdrawal from their duty of attending church. Those who are forced to withdraw by way of hospital admission or are house-bound are remembered during church services with prayer requests for healing.

Churches and worship services provide an environment where people can seek healing. They may accept a diagnosis or a label from a health professional for their deviation from optimum health as they know it but they do not necessarily accept the patient role. According to Parsons, this involves the person actively seeking medical treatment without taking advantage of the sick role. That is, the patient does not always withdraw from their social roles. In seeking spiritual healing the person exhibits a similar approach to that of the person who does not withdraw from their social role but will engage in the additional health enhancing behaviour that health promotion theorists discuss.

The health promotion approach adopted in this thesis does not wholly do away with Parsons' (1975) sick role theory as a description of how and why people behave in modern industrial society when they are sick. Although it is incomplete, we have seen how contemporary sociologists dealing with health issues have used it as a starting point to develop a much expanded model of a broader range of health-seeking behaviour (Weiss and Lonnquist 2005). When they do this, however, we fatally undermine the logical role Parsons' sick role theory played within his broader functionalist theory about the evolutionary change from traditional rural to modern industrial society. Parsons believed that the modern doctor-patient relationship was essential to keep modern industry running by preventing malingering, and that this had created a modern and scientifically governed way of being ill in modern society. Sometimes Parsons is accused by health professionals in training of developing a culturally limited model of the sick role. This rather misses the point; Parsons always thought the sick role was a relatively new development of western industrial society. This eurocentric concept of progress could have contributed to the reasons why contemporary western society has been reluctant to recognise alternative forms of healing and so has been unwilling to legitimise and regulate their practitioners.

Parsons and Lévi-Strauss shared the beliefs of the great majority of sociologists and anthropologists, in the distinction between the primitive and the modern, and that history is the story of the journey from the one to the other. Parsons studied the *modern*, and described the distinctive way in which *modern* people deal with illness as *'the sick role'*. Lévi-Strauss studied the *primitive* mind and described the way *primitive* people deal with illness as *bricolage*. When we turn our minds away from grand theories of history to empirical studies of how people actually behave when they are faced with the never-ending and unavoidable problems of pain, disease and death and an eternity knowable only through faith and speculation, we find remarkable similarities. People do whatever they think will work, and embedded in their assessment of what will work are culturally conditioned rationalities which can be studied, predicted and used to make policy.

Conclusion and Reflections on the Study

The advantages and disadvantages to the researcher of being a member of the same ethnic and cultural group observed and with similar experience of migration to Britain are complex, as noted by Ahmad (1993) and Kelleher (1996). Knowledge of the basic rules and social conduct gave the advantage of easy access to the population but did not necessarily create an ability to interpret the meanings of words and symbols correctly. To observe the relationships between the healer and those requesting healing was interesting although I often felt as if I were an intruder in a sacred space between the participants in their healing relationship and God.

Having access to the community in the researcher's role has highlighted areas of new knowledge, such as the common factors of the power relationships in the hierarchy of the church with the secular world. The fact that there is belief in the authority of the Holy Spirit does not detract from the reality of the human power structures. It is more likely that the authority of the Holy Spirit is acknowledged in words only, rather than be actually appreciated and utilised. I am acutely aware of the complacency of numerous church members in accepting the authority of the Minister, even when they do not agree with the outcomes of such authority. Many do this on the premise that their trust in prayer and in God is not shaken although their trust in the merely human minister may be undermined.

This research has empirically examined the gap between spiritual healing in the churches and the application of health, health promotion, illness and health seeking behaviour models to human behaviour. Theoretically, the importance of religion is acknowledged by the NHS in the appointment of hospital chaplains. Academically, those who research health-seeking behaviour have to accept that *bricolage* is alive and well, and is what ordinary people do with help from a variety of healers. Many church members, however, especially those in the Black majority churches, are not aware of the role of the hospital chaplain. They may have been introduced to the hospital chaplain at the time of illness or death of a family member but nevertheless have failed to notice chaplains and the facilitation they can provide outside church services in terms of sharing prayer and giving pastoral support.

As the ageing population from the "New Commonwealth countries" changes its demography, those becoming ill and nearing death in Britain, and thus having experience of the NHS as a user rather than as an employee, becomes more important. It is therefore incumbent on the statutory health services to make more of an effort to make sure that these elderly people's spiritual as well as physical needs are addressed. This new generational development warrants more research and a closer working with Black majority churches by Health Professionals, supported by NHS funds.

The outcome of the research suggests that seeking spiritual healing as a health seeking behaviour follows the same behavioural models as consultation with health professionals. Despite the differences between them, members of the URC and COGIC congregations feel they experience increased well-being as a result of these activities, and their attitudes and activities can be represented within conventional models of health promotion. In the churches, spiritual healing is a voluntary and free service as there are no medical fees requiring payment through National Insurance or any other scheme. There is no discrimination as healing using touch and anointing with oil is available to all and all are invited for healing whether there is a healing service or not. These factors, as noted in section 1 can make comparison with the efficacy of conventional medical services very difficult.

Some church attenders in both churches hope for the instant fix of a 'miracle' whilst others accept that healing is a slow and ongoing process. Whether it is an instant 'miracle' or an ongoing process, those seeking spiritual healing rely on a belief system and a doctrine that is culturally bound to the Christian faith. These include health promotion activities of prayer, laying on of hands, anointing with oil and also music to effect healing. Recipients of spiritual healing whose health seeking behaviour straddles the medical and the spiritual approaches may or may not use conventional medical services. However in the UK, they usually have the opportunity to access both approaches, unlike people in third world countries who have limited access to modern medicine. They have little or no choice but to make the best use of folk medicine, or faith healers. Nearly twenty years ago Gerloff (1992), writing about both the British and American situations suggested that healing activities could unite black and white worshippers more than any other church activities. In seeking and administering spiritual healing the research reported the researcher contends that individuals and groups are engaging in health seeking behaviour and therefore acknowledging that they are experiencing disease at different levels. These different levels can be integrated in practice.

Once this becomes adequately realised, it becomes the responsibility of health care professionals to involve practitioners of spiritual healing in planning healthcare for their patients. The patient need to be reassured that their health seeking behaviour in terms of spiritual healing is not frowned on by their medical practitioner. When such is the case, a more trusting relationship is established and this will consequently advance both physical and spiritual healing.

There is a clear indication that more research is needed, and that the churches, especially the Black Pentecostals, could familiarize themselves with the discourses and practices of academic research, so that they can present their own contributions fairly and cogently. They can then understand and engage with critiques made by those of other or no faith traditions. Increased interaction between congregations from different ethnic traditions can only improve such understanding.

The access to the research sites and the research subjects enjoyed by the researcher is indicative that members of URC and COGIC congregation and other Christian community might welcome other researchers in action-research approach which will provide some health benefits to the population. It will enable more widely informed health teaching and increasing awareness through health education about health issues such as diabetes, high blood pressure, strokes and sickle cell anaemia which are prominent amongst people who attend black majority churches. Increasing awareness of health and health issues would of course also be valuable amongst people who attend white majority churches.

There is also no reason why the skills of health professionals who are church attenders should not be utilised, if they wish to volunteer to deliver more health education programmes in a church setting. This may be one way of acknowledging that patients who rely on voluntary organisations to meet their cultural, language and specific health needs often do not have the capacity to engage with the statutory organisations such as those directly funded under the National Health Services. Organisations that are funded by tax payers need to take responsibility to seek out voluntary organisations and collaboratively plan health promotion activities to provide the best outcomes for patients and clients. The author has already been involved in health promotion days planned with Pentecostal and Black majority churches alongside health professionals who are also church members and this is done on a voluntary basis. In partnership with the NHS and Church ministers, such planned 'health days', held on church premises where health checks are offered by health professionals from within and outside of the church, should be encouraged and funded by the NHS. These days should be aimed at all ages and families on the same or on separate days. It is important to note that as people live longer there are three—and even more recently four-generation[5] families in the churches as well as in the wider society. Health promotion days therefore could be used as a means of uniting families where either the younger generation or the older generation are regular church attenders. Health checks specific to church attenders should be discouraged as these will encourage segregation instead of integration.

Equally, within NHS health conferences and seminars, the use of prayer and laying on of hands as health promotion activities and health seeking behaviour could be included as demonstration and discussion in the same way as social and voluntary activities around diabetes, sickle cell anaemia, men's health and massage therapy are conducted. This thesis will, it is hoped, add to the knowledge that can assist health promoters in the churches as well as in official Health and Social Care services.

---

[5] Such as that of my superviser, Prof. Thomas Acton, who often worships in the same church with 4 generations of his family present.

References

Achterberg, J., (1985) *Imagery in Healing: Shamanism and Modern Medicine*. Shambala Inc. Boston, Massachusetts.

Acton, T., (1979) ed. Cranford, S."The Gypsy Evangelical Church" *The Ecumenical Review: Journal of the World Council of Churches* Vol.31 (3) pp 279-295.

Acton, T., (2004) *Sociology of Health. Unit code soc 0SOCI0849,* Department of Sociology, University of Greenwich.

Ahmad, W.I.U., (1993) "Making Black people sick: race ideology and health research" in Ahmad, W.I.U., ed. *Race and Health in Contemporary Britain,* Open University Press, Buckingham, pp 11-33.

Ai, A.L., Dunkle, R.E., Peterson, C., and Bolling, S. F., (1998) "The Role of Private Prayer in Psychological Recovery Among Midlife and Aged Patients Following Cardiac Surgery", *The Gerontologist* Vol. 38, pp 591-601.

Albright, C.R., (2000) "The God Module' and the Complexifying Brain." *Journal of Religion and Science* Vol.35 pp. 735-44.

Alder, P., (1975) "The transitional experience: An Alternative view of culture shock".*Journal of Humanistic Psychology* Vol.15 pp. 13-23.

Aldgate, J., and Dimmock, B., (2003) "Managing to Care" in Henderson & Atkinson eds. (2003) pp 3-26.

Al-Krenawi, A., and Graham, J., (1999) "Social Work and Koranic Mental Health Workers" *International Social Work* Vol.42 (1) pp 53-65.

Altheus-Reid, M., (2004) *From Feminist Theology to Indecent Theology*, SCM Press, London.

Anbu, J., (2008) "Developing Intelligent feelings. Improving emotional and social intelligence through education and practice bring benefits at work." *Nursing Standard* Vol. 22 (29) p 52.

Anderson, A., (2004) *An Introduction to Pentecostalism*, Cambridge University Press, Cambridge.

Andrews, D. P., (2002) *Practical Theology for Black Churches*, John Knox Press, Atlanta, Georgia.

Angelo, J., (2002) *Spiritual Healing: Energy medicine for health and wellbeing*, Element Books, London.

Archer, K.J., (2007) "A Pentecostal way of doing Theology: Method and Manner" *International Journal of Systematic Theology*, Vol. 9 (3), pp 301-314.

Armstrong, D., (2001) "The problem of the whole person in holistic medicine" in Davey, Gay and Seale (2002) pp 36-4233-36.

Asher, R., (2002) "Malingering." in Davey, Gay and Seale (2002) pp 170-173.

Atkinson, D., (1991) *The message of Job—Suffering and Grace*. Intervarsity Press, London.

Austin-Broos, D.J. 1992 "Re-defining the moral order—interpretations of Chritianity in post-emancipation Jamaica." in McGlynn F. & Drescher S. eds *The Meaning of freedom: economics, politics, and culture after slavery*, University of Pittsburgh Press, Pittsburgh, pp 221-243.

B.M.A./R.P.S. (British Medical Association and Royal Pharmaceutical Society) (2009) *The British National Formulary*, No.59, British Medical Journal Publishing Group and Pharmaceutical Press, London.

Balarajan, R., Yuen, P., & Raleigh. S., (1989) "Ethnic differences in General practitioner consultation". *British Medical Journal* Vol. 299 pp. 958-960.

Banner R, S., (2001) "Doctoring as a human experience" *Journal of Healing and Caring.* Vol. 1 (1) p1.

Barker, E., (1993) *The Making of a Moonie: Choice or Brainwashing*, Ashgate, London.

Barlow, F., Walker, J., Lewth, G., & Murray, N., (2008) "The experience of spiritual healing" *Journal of Complementary Therapies and Medicine* Vol. 16. pp 223-237.

Barton, J., (1998) *The Cambridge Companion to Biblical Interpretation.* Cambridge University Press, Cambridge.

Battle, M., (2006) *The Black Church in America: African-American Christian Spirituality.* Blackwell, Oxford.

Bazeley, P., & Richards, L., (2000) *The NVivo Qualitative Project Book.* Sage,. London.

Becker, H., (1998) *Tricks of the Trade: How to Think about Your Research While You're Doing It,* University of Chicago Press, Chicago.

Beckford, J., A., & Luckman, T., (1989) *The Changing Face of Religion.*, Sage, London.

Beckford, J., A., (1986) *New Religious Movements and Rapid Social Change,.* Sage, London

Beckford, J.A., (2000) "Religious Movements and Globalization" in Cohen, R., & Rai, S.M., eds. *Global Social Movements*, Athlone Press, London pp.168-183.

Beckford, R., (1998) *Jesus is Dread: Black theology and Black culture in Britain.* Darton, Longman and Todd.

Beckford, R. (2006) *Jesus Dub: Theology, Music and Social Change*, Routledge, London.

Beeghley, L., (2004) 4th edition, *The Structure of Social Stratification in the United States,* University of Florida Press, Gainsville, Florida.

Belcher, J., R., Hall, M., S., (2001) "Healing and Psychotherapy: The Pentecostal Tradition" *Pastoral Psychology* Vol.50(2) pp 63-75.

Benedict, P., (2002) *Christ's Churches Purely Reformed: A Social History of Calvinism*, New Haven, Yale University Press.

Benson, H., Stark, M., (1996) *Timeless Healing: The Power and Biology of Belief,* Scribner, New York.

Bentham, J., (2001ff, originally 1859 ff) *The works of Jeremy Bentham, published under the superintendence of his executor John Bowring,* 11 vols. Elibron Classics, New York.

Berry, J.W., Poortinga, Y. H., Segall, M.H., & Dasen, P.R., (1992) *Cross-cultural Psychology: Research and Application* Cambridge University Press, New York.

Blauner, B., (1990) *Black Lives, White Lives. Three decades of Race Relations in America.* University of California Press, Los Angeles.

Blaxter, M., (1999) "What is Health?" in Davey, Gray and Seale (2002) pp 21-27

Bocock, R., and Thompson. K., eds. (1985) *Religion and Ideology*, Manchester University Press, Manchester.

Boff, C., & Boff, L., (tr. Burns, P.), (1987) *Introducing Liberation Theology*, Orbis, Maryknoll, New York.

Bourguignon, E., (1977) *Spirit Possession.* Chandler and Sharp, San Francisco.

Bowlby, J., (1980) *Attachment and Loss* Vols. 1,2,3, Hogarth, London.

Breslin, M. J., & Lewis, C., A., (2008) "Theoretical models of the nature of prayer and health:. A review" *Mental Health, Religion and Culture.* Vol. 11 (1) pp 9-21.

Brewer, A., (2000) *Ethnography,* Open University Press, Milton Keynes.

Browder, A., T., (1989) *The Browder file: Essays on the African American Experience*, Institute of Karmic Guidance, Washington D.C.

Brown, E., R., Fitzmyer, J. A., & Murphy, R., E., eds. (1996) *The Jerome Biblical Commentary,* Chapman, London.

Bunton, R., & McDonald, G., (1993) *Health Promotion: Disciplines and Diversity*, Routledge, London.

Bury, M., & Gabe, J., (2004) The *Sociology of Health and Illness*, Routledge, London

Byrd, R., C., (1998) "Positive effects of intercessory prayer in a coronary care unit population" *Southern Medical Journal* Vol.87 (7) : pp 826-9.

Calley, M, J, C., (1965) *God's People: West Indian Pentecostal Sects in England.,* Oxford University Press, London.

Campbell, D., (1998) *The Mozart effect: Tapping the power of music to heal, strengthen the mind and unlock the creative spirit.,* Avon, New York, NY

Canavan, D., & Bandon, Y., E., (2005) "Successful treatment of poison oak dermatitis,. Treated with grindelia ssp (gunmead)." *Journal of Alternative and Complementary Medicine.* Vol. 11(4) pp 209-210.

Carr, W., (1989) *The Pastor as Theologian: An Integration of Pastoral Ministry, Theology and Discipleship.*, SPCK, London.

Cassell, E. (1978) *The Healer's Art,.* Penguin Books, Harmondsworth.

Castillo, R.J., (1997) *Culture and mental illness.*, Brooks/Cole, Pacific Grove, CA.

Cipriani, R., (1989) "'Diffused Religion' and New Values in Italy" in Beckford & Luckman (1989) pp 24-48.

Clarke, A., (2001) *The Sociology of Healthcare.* Pearson Education, Harlow

Clebsch, W., A., & Jaekle, C., (1983) *Pastoral Care in a Historical Perspective,* Jason Aronson, Lanham, MD.

Clemmons, I., (1996) *Bishop C.H. Mason and the Roots of the Church of God in Christ,* (Pneuma Life Publishing, Bakersfield, CA).

Coleman, D., (1996) *Emotional Intelligence: Why it can matter more than IQ,* Bloomsbury, London.

Coleman, D., (2006) *Social Intelligence beyond IQ. Beyond Emotional Intelligence: the New Science of Social Relationships* Bantam, New York.

Collinson, P., (2006) *English religion in the age of reformation,.* Continuum International, London.

Constable, T., L., (2008) Notes *on Ephesians.*, Sonic Light Bible Notes, accessed 2008. Note these notes are updated frequently and the current website edition is 2010, at http://www.soniclight.com/constable/notes/pdf/ephesians.pdf. This supersedes the 2008 edition cited.

Cook, J.D., (1981) "The therapeutic use of music: A literature review" *Nursing Forum,* Vol. 20, 252-266.

Copeland, G., (1990) *God's Will is the Holy Spirit,* Kenneth Copeland Publications, Fort Worth, Texas.

Cormick, D., (1998) *Under God's Good hand.: A history of the traditions, which have come together in the URC in the United Kingdom,* United Reformed Church, London.

Coslett, N., (1985) *His Healing Hands,* Marshall Morgan and Scott, Basingstoke.

Cottrell, A., (2005, originally 2000, but updated) *What is Healing Music, a closer look,* The Healing Music Organisation, Santa Cruz, California. http://www.healingmusic.org/Main/What_Is_Healing.htmhttp//www.healingmusic.org.main what is healing?.

Cowley, C., (20095) "Why Medical Ethics should not be taught by Philosophers" *Discourse: Learning and Teaching in Philosophical and Religious Studies* Vol. 51 No 1 pp 50-63. http://www.prs.heacademy.ac.uk/view.html/PrsDiscourseArticles/76.

Creath, K, Schwartz G.E. (2004) "Measuring the effect of music, noise and healing energy" *Journal of Complementary medicine* Vol.10 (1) pp 113-122.

Cross, F, L., Livingstone, E, A., (2000) *The Oxford Dictionary of the Christian Church.* Oxford University Press, London.

Crossman, J., D., (1988, 1999) (Paperback Edition) *The Birth of Christianity. Discovering what happened in the years immediately after the execution of Jesus.* Harper and Collins, New York.

Crowe, B., (2004) "Implications of Technology in Music Therapy; Practice and research for music therapy:. A review of the literature". *Journal of Music Therapy* Vol. 41.(4) pp 282-320 d'Aquili, E and Andrew, N (1999) *The Mystical Mind,* Fortress Books, Minneapolis.

Davey, B., Gray, A., & Seale, C., (2002) *Health and Disease: A Reader.* Open University Press, Buckingham.

Davie, G. Short., C. (19954) *"Church of England General Synod 1990-1995 Analysis of membership" in Davie (1994),* General Synod Papers Series 17, Church House, London.

Davie, G., ed. (1994) *Religion in Britain since 1945: believing without belonging.* Blackwell. Oxford.

Daya, R., (2005) "Buddhist Moments in Psychotherapy" in Moodley & West (2005) pp 182-194.

Denzin, N., (1989) *Sociological Methods: A Source Book,* Prentice Hall, Englewood Cliffs, New Jersey.

Department of Health, (1999) *Saving Lives, Our Healthier Nation,* HMSO, London.

Department of Health, (2000) *The NHS Plan. A Plan for Investment. A Plan for Reform.* HMSO London.

Department of Health, (2002) *The NHS and Community Care Act.* HMSO, London.

Department of Health, (2003a) *Confidentiality. NHS Code of Practice.* HMSO, London.

Department of Health, (2003b) *Reference guide to Consent for Examination and Treatment.* Department of Health and Social Security and Public Safety, HMSO London.

Diamond, J., (1998) *Behavioral Kinesiology,* Harper, New York.

Dickason, C, F., (19953) 2nd Edition *Angels: Elect and Evil,* Christian Research. Institute/Moody Press, Chicago.

Dill, G, B., (20038) *Angel of Music* http//www/geocities.com/Athens/Forum/4225/study24.html accessed 2008, now not available, but transferred to 8 http://www.worshipreleased.com/phpbb/viewtopic.php?f=25&t=110.

Dingwall, R., (1976) *Aspects of Illness* Martin Roberts, London.

Doerkson, B., R., (1996) *Today, Experience Worship,.* C.D. Integrity Music, Mobile, Alabama. (2nd Ed Doerkson, B, R., (2004) *Today: Experience Worship.* CD/DVD, Hosanna Music, Abbotsford, Canada).

Donald, M., (1991) *Origins of the Modem Mind,.* Harvard Univ. Press, Cambridge, Massachusetts.

Dossey, L. (1997) "The return of Prayer" *Alternative Therapies* Vol. 3 (6) pp 10-17.

Dow, J. W., (1986) "Universal Aspects of Symbolic Healing: A Theoretical Synthesis". *American Anthropologist* Vol. 88 pp. 56-69.

Downie, R. S., Fife, C., & Tannahill, A., (1996) *Health Promotion. Models and Values,* Oxford Medical Publications, Oxford.

Dubos, R., (1995) "Mirage of Health" in Davey, Gray and Seale (2002) pp 4-9.

Durkheim, E. *(*1954, originally 1912*) The Elementary Forms of Religious Life*, Allen and Unwin, London.

Ehrenreich, B., (1989) *The Inner Life of the Middle Class,.* Harper-Collins, New York.

Ela, Jean-Marc, (1994) "Christianity and Liberation in Africa," in Gibellini, R ed. *Paths of African Theology,* Orbis Books, Maryknoll, New York pp 136-50.

Elgood, C., (1934) *Medicine in Persia,*. Paul B Hoeber Inc., New York.

Erez, M., & Gati, E., (2004) "A Dynamic, multi-level Model of Culture. From the Micro level of individual to the Macro level of a global Culture" *Applied Psychology: An International Review* Vol.53(4) pp 583-598.

Etherington, M., (2003) *The Antigua & Barbuda Companion,* Interlink Books, New York.

Ewles, L., & Simnett, I. (2003, 2005) *Theories of Health Promotion and Health Education:A Practical Guide to Health Educatio, n.* Bailliere Tindall,. Edinburgh.

Ewles, L., & Simnett, I., (1999) *Promoting Health. A Practical Guide to Health Education.* Harcourt, Edinburgh.

Feierman, S., & Janzen, J., (eds), 1992 *The Social Basis of Health and Healing in Africa,* University of California Press, Berkeley.

Fleischman, P. R., (1990) *The Healing Spirit:. Case Studies in Religion and Psychotherapy,* SPCK, London.

Foster, F., & Foster, R., (1987) "Women's spiritual gifts in the church" in Keay (1987).

Frecska, E., & Zsuanne, K., (1989) "Social Bonding in the Modulation of the Physiology of Ritual Trance". *Ethos* Vol. 1 (1) pp 70-87.

Gaunton, C., E., (1997) *The Cambridge Companion on Christian Doctrine.*, Cambridge University Press, Cambridge.

Geissmann, T (1999) "Gibbon Songs and Human Music from an Evolutionary Perspective" in N. Wallin, B. Merker, and S. Brown (eds), (1999).

Gibellini, R., (1994) *Paths of African Theology,* Orbis, Maryknoll, New York.

Gilbert, D. (2002) 6th edition *The American Class Structure in an Age of Growing Inequality,*. Wadsworth, Belmont, California.

Gill, R., (1996) "Discourse Analysis: Practical Implications" in Richardson (1996).

Glaser, B., and Strauss, A., (1967) *The discovery of grounded theory,* Aldine Publications, Chicago.

Godfrey, W., R., (2002) "Evangelical or Reformed" *New Horizon, Journal of the Orthodox Presbyterian Church,* April, http://www.opc.org/nh.html?article_id=193http:/www.opc.org/new-horizon/NH02/02e.html.

Goffman, E., (1968,) (New Edition) *Asylums,* Pelican, Harmondsworth.

Goffman, E., (1969) "The Insanity of Place" *Journal for the Study of Interpersonal Processes.* Vol32 (4), (also in Davey, Gray & Seale, (2002) pp 82-85).

Goldman, A., I., (1993) *Readings in Philosophy and Cognitive Science.,* MIT press, Cambridge, Massachussetts.

Gooch, S., (2007) "Save your prayers" *Nursing Standard* Vol. 22 (no. 11) pp 20-21 Nov 2007.

Good, B., (1994) *Medicine, Rationality and Experience: An Anthropological Perspective,* Cambridge University Press, New York and Cambridge.

Good, C.M., Hunter, J.M., Katz, S.H., and Katz, S.S., (1979) "The interface of dual systems of health care in the developing world: Toward health policy initiatives in Africa" *Social Science and Medicine,* Vol. 13, pp 141-154.

Gottwald, N., K., (1999) *The Tribes of Yahweh: sociology of the religion of liberated Israel.* Sheffield Academic Press, Sheffield.

Gottwald, N., K., (1989) "The Exodus as an Event and Process: A test case in the Biblical Grounding of Liberation Theology" in Ellis, M.H., and Madiro, O., (1989) *The Future of Liberation Theology*, Orbis Books, Maryknoll, N.Y.

Graham, H., (1999) *Complementary Therapies in Context: The psychology of healing*, Jessica Kingsley, Bristol and London.

Gran, P (1979) "Medical Pluralism in Arab and Egyptian History" *Social Science and Medicine* Vol. 13 (4): pp. 339-348.

Greenwood, B., (1992) "Cold or spirits? Ambiguity and syncretism in Moroccan therapeutics" in Feierman & Janzen (eds), (1992) pp. 285-314.

Guthrie, S, R., (2003) "Singing in the body and in the Spirit." *Journal of the Evangelical Theological Society*. Vol. 46 (4) pp. 633-46.

Hall, S., (1985) "Religious Ideology and Social Movements in Jamaica" in. Bocock and Thompson. (1985) pp 269-296.

Hallett, A., (2004) "Narratives of Therapeutic Touch". *Nursing Standard* vol. 19. (1) pp 33-37.

Hammersley, M., & Atkinson, P., (1992, 2007) *Ethnography. Principles and practice*. Routledge, Basingstoke.

Hammersley, M., (1993) *What's Wrong with Ethnography?* Routledge, London.

Hannen, S., (2003) *Healing by design: Unlocking your body's potential to heal itself*, Strang/Siloam Books, Lake Mary, Florida.

Hanser, S. B., (1990) "A music therapy strategy for depressed older adults in the community". *The Journal of Applied Gerontology*, Vol. 9 No (. 3), pp. 283-98.

Hanser, S, B., (2005a) "Effects of music therapy intervention for women with metastatic breast cancer". *Oncology Nursing Forum* Vol. 31 (1) pp 20-25.

Harris, P., (2002) *Sermon on Mark 1:29-39*, First Christian Church of Melbourne, Florida. (Disciples of Christ) http://www.fcc/bournere.org/Rev.%20Harris%20Sermon.htm Accessed 12/9.2006.

Harrison, S. (2004) "Music reduces stress levels amongst staff and patients". *Nursing Standard* Vol. 18 (30) p 4.

Hart, D (1969) *Bisayan Philipino and Malayan Humoral Pathologies: Folk Medicine and Ethnohistory in South East Asia.* South East Asia Program, Data Paper No. 76. Ithaca: Dept. of Asian Studies, Cornell University, Ithaca.

Harvey, A, E., (2004) *A Companion to the New Testament.* Cambridge University Press, Cambridge.

Harvey, P., (2005) *Freedom's coming: religious culture and the shaping of the South from the Civil War through the civil rights era,* University of North Carolina Press, Chapel Hill, North Carolina.

Hawley, G., & Irurita, V., (1998) "Seeking Comfort through prayer" *International Journal of Nursing Practice* Vol. 4 pp 9-18.

Hayter, M., (1987) *The New Eve in Christ,* SPCK, London.

Helman, C.G, (2002) "Feed a cold, starve a fever" in Davey, Gray and Seale (2002) pp 14-20.

Helman, C.G. ed. (2001) (4th ed) *Culture, Health and Illness* E. Arnold, London.

Henderson, J. &, Atkinson, D. eds. (2003) *Managing Care in Context,* Routledge, London.

Hewitt-Taylor, J., (2001) "Use of constant comparative analysis in qualitative research" *Nursing Standard* Vol.5 (42) pp 39-42.

Hickey, M., (2000) *Breaking the Generational Curse*, Marilyn Hickey Ministries/Harrison House, Tulsa Oklahoma.

Hill, M., & Zwaga, W., (1989) "Religion in New Zealand. Changes and Comparison" in Beckford & Luckman 1989.

Hill, M., (1973) *A Sociology of Religion*, Heinemann Educational Books, London.

Hiro, D., (1991) *Black British, White British, A History of Race Relations in Britain*, Collins, London.

Holland, K., & Hogg, C., (2001) *Cultural Awareness in Nursing and Health Care: An introductory text*, E.Arnold, London.

Hollenweger, W, J., (1972) *The Pentecostals: The Charismatic Movements in the Churches*, Augsburg, and Minneapolis.

Hollenweger, W, J., (1973) "Pentecostalism and Black Power" *Theology Today* 30 (3) pp 228-238.

Holmes, T. H. & Rahe, R.H. (1967) "The Social Readjustment Scale." *Journal of Psychosomatic Research* Vol.11 pp.213-218.

Home Office, (2000a) *Race Relations (Amendment) Act*, The Stationery Office London

Home Office, (2000b) *Human Rights Act: An introduction*, Home Office Communications Directory, London.

Hughes, C., (1997) "Prayer and Healing", *Journal of Holistic Nursing* Vol 15. (3) pp 318-324.

Hummel, C., & Hummel, A., (1990) *Spiritual Gifts*, Intervarsity Press, London. See also Stevens 2004, a later edition.

Hunter, J., Anderson, K., (2008) "Respiratory Assessment" *Nursing Standard.* Vol. 22. pp 41-43.

Hutson, S, R., (2000) "The rave: spiritual healing in modern western subcultures" *Anthropological Quarterly*, Vol. 73 (1) pp 35-4.9

Idler, E.L (1995) "Religion, Health, and Nonphysical Senses of Self" *Social Forces* Vol. 74, pp 683-704.

Illich I., (1976) *Limits to Medicine: Medical Nemesis, the Expropriation of Health*, Marian Boyars, London.

Ingliss, B., (1980) *Natural medicine*, Fontana/Collins, Glasgow.

Jagessar, M.N., & Reddie, A. G., eds. (2007) *Post-Colonial Black British Theology: New Textures and Themes*, Epworth Press, Peterborough.

James, M., (2002) "Hysteria and Demonic possession" in Davey et al eds. (2002) pp 44-50

Janzen, J.M., (1992) "Preface" in Feierman and Janzen eds., (1992).

Jaye, C., (2001) "Explaining suffering and healing: A comparison of Pentecostal and secular general practitioners" *NZFP New Zealand Family Practitioner* Vol. 23 (5) p 23.

Jeffries, I., (2003) *Managing Care at Wellbridge*, Open University CD Rom, Milton Keynes.

Johnson, M., (2008) "Can compassion be taught?" *Nursing Standard.* Vol. 23 (1) pp 19-21.

Jones, N., (2002) *The English Reformation: Religious and Cultural Adaptation*, Blackwell, Oxford.

Jones, R., (1980) *Groundwork of worship and preaching*, Epworth Press, Peterborough.

Jules-Rosette, B., (1989) "The new religion of Africa" in Beckford & Luckman (1989) pp 147-162.

Jung, C.G., ed. Violet S. de Laszlo, (1959) *The Basic Writings of C.G. Jung*, The Modern Library, New York.

Kasl, S., and Cobb, S., (1966) "Health Behavior, Illness Behavior", and "Sick Role Behavior: A review" *Archives of Environmental Health*. Vol. 12 (2) 246–266. and Vol. 12 (4) 531-541

Katz, J. J., (1990) *Metaphysics of Meaning*, MIT Press, Cambridge, Massachusetts.

Kaufman, G., (1996) *The Psychology of Shame, Theory and treatment of Shame-Based Syndromes*, Routledge, London.

Keay, K., ed., (1987) *Men Women and God: Evangelicals on Feminism*, Marshall Pickering, Basingstoke.

Kee, A., (2006) *The Rise and Demise of Black Theology*, Ashgate, London.

Keighley, T, (2007) "Body and Soul". *Nursing Standard*. Vol 22 (9) pp 20-21

Kelleher, D. (1996) "A defence of the use of the terms 'ethnicity' and 'culture'" in Kelleher, D. and Hillier, S. eds. (1996) *Researching Cultural Differences in Health*, Routledge. London, pp 69-90.

Kelly, M., (1992) *Colitis*, Routledge, London & New York.

Kendal-Raynor, P., (2008) "Undervalued and under threat: NHS Chaplains feel the pressure" *Nursing Standard* vol. 25 (34) p 10.

King, E., (2002) "The use of self in qualitative research" in Richardson J. T., ed., (2002 2nd Edition) *Handbook of Qualitative Research Methods for Psychologists and the Social Sciences*, The British Psychological Society/Blackwell, Oxford, pp 175-188.

King, G., (1976) *You too can heal*, Aetherius Press, London.

Kirkpatrick, L., (1997) "An Attachment-Theory Approach to Psychology of Religion" in Spilka, B. and McIntosh, D.N. and Daniel, M. (eds), *The Psychology of Religion: Theoretical Approaches*, Westview, Boulder, Colorado, pp 114-33.

Koehn, D., (1994) *The Groundwork of Professional Ethics*. Routledge, London.

Koss-Chioino, J. D., (2005) "Spirit healing, mental health and emotion regulation" *Zygon* 40 (2) pp 409-422.

Kramsch, C., (1998) *Language and Culture*, Oxford University Press, Oxford.

Krieger, D., (1975) "Therapeutic Touch: The imprimatur of Nursing" *American Journal of Nursing* Vol. 75 pp. 784-787.

Krieger, D., Peper, E., Ancoli, S., (1979) "Therapeutic Touch: Seraching for evidence of Physiological Change" *American Journal of Nursing* Vol.79 (4) pp 660-662.

Krucoff, M. W., Crater, S.W., Gallup, D., Blankenship, J.C., Cuffe, M., Guaneri, M., Krieger R.A., Kshettry, V.R., Morris, K., Oz, M., Pichard, A., Sketch, M.H., Koenig, H.G., Mark, D., & Lee, K.L., (2005) "Music, imagery touch and prayer as adjunct to interventional cardiac care" *The Lancet* Vol. 366 pp. 211-17.

Kuhn, T.S., 1970 *The Structure of Scientific Revolutions*, University of Chicago Press, Chicago.

Lai, Y.M., (1999) "Effects of music listening on depressed women in Taiwan" *Issues in Mental Health Nursing* Vol. 20 (3) pp 229-46.

Lambert, N., Barlow, F., Walker, J., Lewth, G., Murray, N., (2008) "The experience of Spiritual Healing" *Journal of Complementary Medicine* Vol.16 pp 223-237.

Laming, Lord / The Home Office (2003) *The Victoria Climbie Inquiry Report* Cm. 5730, TSO (The Stationery Office), London.

Lamont, S., (1989) *Church and State: Uneasy Alliances*, Mackays, Chatham. Kent.

Langley, M., (1987) "The ordination of Women" in Keay (1987) pp 80-81.

Larco, L., (1997) "Encounters with the Huacas: ritual dialogue, music and healing in Northern Peru" *The World of Music,* Vol. 39 (1) pp. 35-59.

Lawrence, R., (2001) *The Magic of Healing,* Thorsons, London.

Leininger, M., and McFarland (1997, 2002) *Transcultural Nursing: Concepts, Theories, Research and Practices,* McGraw-Hill, New York.

Levenstein, S., (1998) "Stress and Peptic Ulcer: Life beyond helicobacter" *British Medical Journal* Vol. 316, (14th Feb), p 538.

Levin, J. S., & Schiller, P. L., (1987) "Is there a religious factor in health?" *Journal of Religion and Health* Vol. 26 pp 9-36.

Lévi-Strauss, C., (1966) *The Savage Mind,* University of Chicago Press, Chicago.
Lévi—Strauss, C., (1963) "The effectiveness of Symbols" in Lévi—Strauss, C., (1963) *Structural Anthropology,* Penguin, Harmondsworth pp 186-205.

Lewis, C, S., (2003, originally 1940) *The Problem of Pain,* Harper Collins, New York.

Linnett, P., (2005) "Finding a place in a dislocated world: reflections on depression" *Spirituality and Health.* Vol. 6 (1) pp 43-50.
Littlewood, R., Dein, S., eds. (2000) *Cultural Psychology and Medical Anthropology: An Introduction and Reader,* Athlone Press, London.

Lowdell, C., (2000) *Health of Ethnic Minority Elders in London,* The Health of Londoners Project, London.

Lucas, E., ed., (1997) *Christian Healing: What can we believe?* Lynx Communications, London.

Lynch, T., (2004) *Beyond Prozac: Healing Mental Health Suffering without drugs,* Mercier, Cork.

MacKenzie, R. A. F., & Murphy, R. E., 1996 "Job" in Brown et al (1996).

Macrae, J., (1988) *Therapeutic Touch: A practical guide,* Knopf, New York.

Marris, P., (1974, 1986) *Loss and Change,* Routledge & Kegan Paul, London.

Martin, D., & Hill, M. eds. (1970) *A Sociological Yearbook of Religion in Britain,* SCM Press, London.

Marx, K. & Engels F. (New Edition) 2008 *On Religion* Dover Books, New York.

MacRobert, I., (1988) *The Black Roots and White Racism of Early Pentecostalism in the USA,* Macmillan, New York.

Mbiti, J., (1969) *African religion and philosophy,* Heinemann African Writers Series, Nairobi. London.

McAdams, D, P., & West, S, G., (1997) "Introduction: Personality, Psychology and the case study" *Journal of Personality* Vol 65 (4) 757-785.

McGovern, A, F., (1989) *Liberation Theology and its Critics: Towards an assessment,* Orbis Maryknoll, N.Y.

McCollough, M., (1995) "Prayer and Health: Conceptual Issues, Research Review and Research Agenda" *Journal of Psychology and Theology* Vol. 23 (1) pp 15-29.

McCracken, G.D., (1988) *The Long Interview*, Sage, London.

McGrath, A. E., (1995) *The Christian Theology Reader*, Blackwell, Oxford.

Mercandetti, M., & Cohen A.J., (2008) *Wound Healing and Repair*, Department of Surgery. Hospital of Sarasota. USA. eMedicine from WebMD, http://emedicine.medscape.com/article/1298129-overview.

Merker, B., (2000) "Synchronous Chorusing and Human Origins" in Wallin, Merker, and Brown, eds., (2000) pp 315-327.

Meyers, J.,(1995) *Battlefield of the Mind: Winning the battle in your mind*, Thomas Nelson Inc., St.Louis, Missouri.

Miles, M. B., & Huberman, A. M., (1994) *Qualitative Data Analysis*, Sage, London & New York.

MIMS (2007) *MIMS for Nurses Independent Prescriber Formulary* Haymarket Publications, London.

Molino, J., (1999) 'Toward an Evolutionary Theory of Music', in Wallin, Merker, and Brown, eds., (1999) pp 165-76.

Moltman, J., (1997) *The Source: The Holy Spirit and the Theology of Life*, SCM Press, and London.

Moodley, R., & West, W., (2005) *Integrating traditional healing practices into Counselling and Psychotherapy*, Sage, London.

Morris, J, N., (2001)" Pride against Prejudice: Lives not Worth Living", in Davey, Gray and Seale eds. (2002) pp 118 – 121.

Moyer, C. A., James, R., & Hannan, J, W., (2004). "A Meta Analysis of Massage Therapy Research" *American Psychological Journal* Vol. 130 (1) pp 13-18.

Muddiman, J., New Edition (2004) *Epistle to the Ephesians: Black's New Testament Commentary.* Baker Academic, Grand Rapids, Michigan.

Mulkay, M., (1991) *Sociology of Science: A Sociological Pilgrimage*, Open University Press, Milton Keynes.

Muncey, T., (2010) *Creating Auto-ethnographies*, Sage, New York.

Munroe, M., (2001) *Understanding the purpose and power of prayer: Earthly license for heavenly interference*, Faith Ministries International, Nassau.

Murray-Parkes, C., (1986) *Bereavement: Studies of Grief in Adult life.* Pelican, Harmondsworth.

Muser, D. W., & Price, J. L., (1992) *A New Handbook of Christian Theology*, Lutterworth Press, Cambridge.

Myss, C., (1997) *Anatomy of the Spirit: The Seven Stages of Power and Healing*, Bantam Books, London.

Narayanasamy, A., & Narayanasamy, M., (2008) "The healing power of prayer and its implications for nursing" *British Journal of Nursing* Vol. 17 (6) pp 394-398.

Neal, E. G., (1972) *The Healing Power of Christ*, Hodder and Stoughton, London.

Norman, A., (1985) "Triple Jeopardy: The Centre on Policy for Ageing" in Holland and Hogg (2001).

Novella, S., (1998) "The Touch of Life" *New England Journal of Skeptism* Vol. 1 (4) pp 12-24.

O'Laoire, S., (1997) "An experimental study of the effects of Distant Intercessory Prayer on Self Esteem and Depression" *Alternative Therapies* Vol.3 (6) pp 38-53.

Oakley, A., (1995) "Doctor Knows Best" in Davey, Gray and Seale eds. (2002) pp 357-362.

Oduyoye, M, A., (1994) "Feminist Theology in an African Perspective" in Gibellini 1994 pp 166-180.

Oppenheimer, M. (2011) *Articles exposing the false gospel of Kenneth Copeland* http://www.deceptioninthechurch.com/kcopeland.html Accessed 21 January 2011.

Osterman, E. V., (1998) *What God says about music.* AWSAHM Music, Huntsville, Alabama.

Owour, O. B., Oketch-Rabah, H., Kokward, J. O., (2006) "Rejuvenating therapeutic fellowships: The jolang'o in Luo African independent churches" *Mental Health, Religion and Culture* Vol. 9 (5) pp 423-434.

Packer, J. I., Nystrom, C., (2006) *Praying, Finding our way from Duty to Delight*, Intervarsity Press, London.

Paris, J. P., (1985) *The Social Teaching of the Black Churches*, Fortress Publications, Philadephia.

Parkes, C. M., 2nd Edition (1986) *Bereavement: Studies of Grief in Adult Life*, Tavistock/Pelican, London.

Parsons, T., (1951) *The Social System*, Free Press of Glencoe, New York.

Parsons, T., (1975) "The Sick Role and the role of the Physician reconsidered" *Health and Society* Vol. 53 pp 257-278.

Paterson, P., (2006) "Do we believe in Miracles? The miracles of Jesus" *Daily Mail* August 7th p 9.

Patte, D., (1995) *The Ethics of Biblical Interpretation: A Re-evaluation*, Westminster John Knox Press, Louisville, Kentucky.

Patterson, N., (2008) "Caring for patients after death" *Nursing Standard* Vol. 22. (51) pp 48-56.

Pearce P. L., (2005) *Aspects of Tourist Behaviour: Themes and Conceptual Schemes*, Channel View, Bristol.

Peters, S., F., (2008) *When prayer fails: Faith Healing, Children and the Law* Oxford University Press, London.

Phillips, R. L., & Snowdown D., (1983) *Association of Meat and Coffee use with Cancers of the Large Bowel, Breast and Prostate among Seventh Day Adventists*, Paper presented at Conference on Nutrition in Cancer Causation and prevention, Loma Linda University, California.

Phillips, R. L., Kumza, J.W., Beeson L.W., & Lotz T., (1980) "Influence of selection versus lifestyle on risk of Fatal Cancer and Cardiovascular Disease among Seventh—Day Adventists" *American Journal of Epidemiology* Vol. 112 (2) pp 296-314.

Pinto, T.O., (1997) "The Healing process: a musical drama: the Ebo ceremony in the Bahian Candomble of Brazil" *The World of Music* Vol. 39 (1 pp. 11-33.

Poloma, M.M., & Pendleton, B.F., (1991) 'The Effects of Prayer and Prayer Experiences on Measures of General Well-Being' *Journal of Psychology and Theology*, Vol. 19 pp 71-83.

Popper, K., (2002) *The Logic of Scientific Discoveries*, Routledge Classics, London.

Posner, G. P., (1995) "Florida Woman's 'miraculous' cure" *Skeptical Inquirer* Vol.19 http://members.aol.com/garypos/miraculous.cure.html.

Priestley, M., (1975) *Music Therapy in Action*, Constable, London.

Prince, R., (1982) "The Endorphins: A Review for Psychological Anthropologists" *Ethos* Vol. 10 (4) pp 299-302.

Pullar, P., (1988) *Spiritual and Lay Healing,* Penguin, Harmondsworth.

Quinn, J. P., (1989a) "Future directions of therapeutic research" *Journal of Holistic Nursing* Vol. 7 (1) pp 19-25.

Quinn, J. P., (1989b) "Therapeutic touch as energy exchange replication and extension." *Nursing Science Quarterly* Vol. 2 (2) pp 79-87.

Quinn, J., P (1984) "Therapeutic Touch as energy exchange: Testing the theory".*Advances in Nursing Science* Vol.6 (1) pp. 37-45.

Radford Reuther, R., (1983) *Sexism and God talk: Towards a Feminist Theology,* SCM Press, and London.

Rahner, K., (1982) *The practice of faith: A handbook of contemporary spirituality.* SCM Press, London.

Raleigh, S., & Balarajan, R., (1994) "Public health and the 1991 census" *British Medical Journal* Vol. 309 p 287.

Ralph, S., Adams, J., & Atkinson, D., (2003) "Taking account of History", in Henderson, J., and Atkinson, D. eds.,(2003) *Managing Care in Context,* Routledge, London, pp 283-308.

Rauscher, F., Shaw, G., & Ky, K., (1993) "Music and spatial performance" *Nature* Vol. 365 p 611.

Rayburn, C., and Richmond, L., eds. (2002) "Theobiology: Interfacing Theology, Biology and the Other Sciences for Deeper Understanding" *American Behavioral Scientist* Special Number, Vol. 45 (12) pp 1785-1912.

Rehman, F., (1989) *Health and Medicine in Islamic Tradition,* The Crossroad Publishing Company, New York.

Reynolds, J., Seden, J., (2003) *Managing Care in Practice*, Open University Press, Milton Keynes.

Rice, H.L., & Huffstattler, J.C., (2001) *Reformed Worship*, Geneva Press, Louisville, Kentucky.

Richards, L., (1999) *Using NVivo in qualitative research,*. Sage, London.

Richardson A., & Bowden, J., (1999) *A New Dictionary of Christian Theology*, SCM Press, London.

Richardson, J.T., (1996) *Handbook of Qualitative Research Methods for Psychology and the Social Sciences*, British Psychological Society, Leicester.

Riggs, M. Y., (1994) *Arise Awake and Act: A Womanist Call for Black Liberation*, Pilgrims Press, Cleveland, Ohio.

Robbins, D. A., (1995) *What people say about the Church*, Victorious Publications, Grass Valley, California.

Roberts, L., Ahmed, I., Hall, S., & Davison, A, (2009) "Intercessory prayer for the alleviation of ill health" *Cochrane Database of Systematic Reviews*, Issue 2. Art. No.: CD000368. DOI: 10.1002/14651858.CD000368.pub3 http://www2.cochrane.org/reviews/en/ab000368.html.

Robertson, R., (1972) *Sociology of Religion*, Penguin, Baltimore

Rogers, A., & Reynolds, J., (2003) "Leadership and Vision" in Reynolds and Seden (2003) pp 57-82.

Rogers, C. R., (1990) *Client Centered Therapy*, Constable, London.

Roper, N., Logan, W.W & Tierney, A.J., (2000) *The Roper-Logan-Tierney Model of Nursing: Based on Activities of Living*, Elsevier Health Sciences. Edinburgh.

Rosato, P.J., (1999) "The Holy Spirit" in Richardson & Bowden (1999) pp 262-269.

Rose, F. G., (1999) "Ethnic minority elders! Who cares? Health and social care needs of black and ethnic minority elders by the statutory services". *Journal of Managing Clinical Nursing.* vol.1 (1) pp 111-115.

Rose, F.G., (2002) "A spoonful of sugar does not make the medicine goes down. Questions and answers on Diabetes amongst African Caribbean people" *Focus Journal, The magazine of the African and Caribbean Evangelical Alliance.* Autumn Issue p 9.

Rose, F. G., (2003) "Is your blood boiling?" *Focus Journal, The magazine of the African and Caribbean Evangelical Alliance.* Spring Issue. P 9.

Roseman, M., (1991) *Healing sounds from the Malaysian rainforest: Temiar music and medicine,* University of California Press, Berkeley, CA.

Rottschaefer, W., (1999) "Philosophical and Religious Implications of Cognitive Social Learning Theories of Personality" *Zygon* Vol. 26 pp 137-48.

Rowanchilde, R., (19972003) *A Time for prayer,* Salaam Canada http://www.salaamcanada.org/study7.html.

Samson, C., (1999) *Health Studies: A Critical and Cultural Reader,* Blackwell, Oxford.

Sayre-Adams, J., & Wright, S.G., (1995) *Therapeutic Touch: Theory and Practice,* Churchill Livingstone, New York.

Schaff, P., 3rd. ed. (2006) *History of the Christian Church,* 8 Vols. Hendrickson, Peabody, Massachusetts.

Schlitz, M., Braud, W., (1997) "Distant Intentionality and Healing: Assessing the Evidence" Journal *of Alternative Therapies* Vol.3 (6) pp 62-73.

Schneider, R.H., Staggers F., Alexander C. N., Sheppard W., Rainforth M., & Konwani, K., (1995) "A randomised controlled trial of stress reduction for hypertension in older African Americans", *Hypertension*, 26(5) pp. 820-827.

Schwartz, G.E., (2004) "Measuring the effects of music, noise and healing energy using a seed germination". *Journal of Complementary Medicine and therapy.* Vol.10 (1) pp. 113-22.

Seale, C., & Filmer P., (1998) "Doing Social Surveys" in Clive Seale Ed. (1998) *Researching Society and Culture,* Sage, London.

Seedhouse, D., (1997) *Health Promotion: Philosophy, Prejudice and Practice,* John Wiley & Sons, London & New York.

Sheldon, L., (1998) "Grounded Theory:. Issues for Research in Nursing" *Nursing Standard* Vol. 12 (552) pp 47-50.

Siegel, R. E., (1968) *Galen's System of Physiology and Medicine,* S. Karger, Basel.

Sieh, A., & Brentin., L. K., (1997) *The Nurse Communities.* W.B. Saunders, Philadelphia.

Snowdown, D. A., & Phillips, R.L., (1984) *Diet in the Etiology of Breast Cancer,* Elsevier, New York.

Spry, T., (2001) "Performing auto-ethnography: An embodied methodological praxis" *Qualitative Enquiry,* Vol. 7 (6) pp 706-732.

Stacey, J., (1977) *Groundwork of Theology,* The Garden City Press, London.

Stacey, M., (1986) "Concepts of Health and Illness and the Division of Labour in Health Care" in Currer C. & Stacey M. eds., *Concepts of Health, Illness and Disease: A Comparative Perspective,* Berg, Oxford.

Stacey, M., (1988) *Sociology of Health and Illness,* Unwin Hyman, London.

Stacy, R., Brittain, K., & Kerr, S., (2002) "Singing for Health: an exploration of the issues" *Health Education.* Vol. 102 (4) pp 156-162.

Steel, M., (2005) *Pentecostalism in Zambia: Power, Authority and the Overcomers. An examination of the growth and effects of Pentecostalism on development,* M.Sc Dissertation, University of Wales.

Stephanides, S. L., & Moore C., (2009) "Plant Poison, Toxicodendron." *eMedicine from WebMD* http://emedicine.medscape.com/article/817671-overview.

Stevens, R.P., (2004) *Spiritual Gifts,* Scripture Union, London. Note: this is a later edition of Hummel and Hummel (1990).

Stolley, J., Buckwalter, K., & Koenig, H., (1999) "Prayer and religious coping for caregivers of persons with Alzheimer's disease and related disorders" *American Journal of Alzheimer's Disease and Related Disorders* Vol.14 (3) pp 181-191.

Sully, P., & Dallas, J., (2005) *Essential Communication Skills for Nursing,* Elsevier, London.

Sundar, S., (2005) "Effects of music therapy and counselling: A state of anxiety of Ca-hypo-pharynx patients" *Music Therapy Today* Vol. 7 (1) pp 8-29.

Swearinigen, P. P., (2006) 6th Edition *A Manual of Medical-Surgical Nursing care, Nursing Interventions and Collaborative Management,* Mosby Books, St Louis, Missouri.

Swenson, K., M., (2005) *Living through Pain: Psalms and the search for wholeness,* Baylor University Press, Waco, Texas.

Tambiah, S, J., (1990) *Magic, Science, Religion, and the Scope of Rationality*, Cambridge University Press, Cambridge.

Tantam, D., (1993) "An exorcism in Zanzibar: insights into groups from another culture" *Group Analysis* Vol. 26 pp. 251-260.

Targ, E., Thomson, K. S., (1997) "Research in distant healing intentionality is feasible and deserves a place on out national research agenda" *Alternative Therapies* Vol. 3 (6) pp 92-96.

Taylor, S., (2002) *Ethnographic Research: A Reader*, Sage, London.

Temkin, O., (1973) *Galenism: Rise and Decline of a Medical Philosophy*, Cornell University Press, Ithaca, NY.

Teuton, J., Dowrick, C., & Bentall, R., P., (2007) "How healers manage the pluralistic healing context: The perspective of psychosis in religious and allopathic healers in relation to psychosis in Uganda" *Social Science and Medicine*, Vol. 65 (6) pp 1260-1273.

Thomas-Juggan, N., (2000) *The Story of the Calvary Church of God in Christ in England. History, Organization, Structure and Doctrine*, Minerva Press, London.

Thorogood, N., (1993) "What is the Relevance of Sociology for Health Promotion" in Bunton and McDonald (1993).

Tomatis, A. A., (1991) *The Conscious Ear*, Station Hill Press, Barrytown, N.Y.

Torres, L.R., & Torres, C. A., (1998) *Notes on Music*, TorresLC Ministries, Gaston, Oregon.

Toulis, N.R. (1997) *Believing Identity: Pentecostalism and the Mediation of Jamaican Ethnicity*, Berg, Oxford.

Troeltsch, E., (*1931*) *The Social Teaching of the Christian Churches,* George Allen and Unwin, London:

Tugwell, S., Hocken, P., Every, G., & Mills, J., (1976) *New Heaven, New Earth: An encounter with Pentecostalism.* Darton, Longman & Todd, London.

Tutu, D., (1986) *Crying in the Wilderness,* Mowbray, Oxford.

Twigg, J. (1979), "Food for thought: purity and vegetarianism" *Religion,* Vol. 9 (1) pp.13-35.

United Reformed Church General Assembly (1982) *Seven Fundamental Qualifications for Ministry.* http://www.urc.org.uk/what_we_do/the_manual/ministries#fundamental_qualifications

United Reformed Church, (1989) *URC Service Book*, URC, London.

United Reformed Church, (2008) *Yearbook.* URC, London.

Valle, J., Raymond, P., (1989) "Religious Experience as Self Healing Mechanisms". in Ward, C., ed., (1989), *Altered States of Consciousness and Mental Health: A Cross Cultural Perspective*, Sage, San Francisco, California, pp 149-66.

Vaskilampi, T., Hanninen, O., (1982) "Cupping as a Traditional Healing Treatment in Eastern Finland" in Vaskilampi, T., & MacCormack, C.P., eds., (1982) *Folk Medicine and Health Culture: The Role of Folk Medicine in Modern Health Care.*, The University of Koupio Department of Public Health, Koupio, Finland.

Village, A., (2005) "Dimensions of belief about miraculous healing", *Mental Health Religion and Culture* Vol. 8 (2) 97-107.

Wagner, C. P., (1992) *Prayer Shield*, Monarch, Tunbridge Wells.

Waine, B., & Henderson, J., (2003), "Managers, managing and managerialism", in Henderson and Atkinson, (2003) pp 49-74.

Wainwright, D., Calnan, M., (2002) *Work Stress: The Making of a Modern Epidemic*, Open University Press, Milton Keynes.

Waldfogel, S., (1997) "Spirituality in Medicine" in Randall J.R., & Lazar, J.S., eds., *Complementary and Alternative Therapies in Primary Care,* Primary Care Series, Vol. 24 (4), W.B.Saunders, Philadelphia pp 963-974.

Walkert, T. (2004) *Mothership Connections A Black Atlantic Synthesis of Neoclassical Metaphysics and Black Theology,* SUNY Press, New York.

Wallin, N., Merker, B. and Brown, S., eds. (1999) *The Origins of Music,* MIT Press, Cambridge, Massachussetts.

Walter, T., (1994) *The Revival of Death.* Routledge, London.

Walsh, D., (2001) "Doing Ethnography" in Seale, C., Ed. *Researching Society and Culture,* Sage, London.

Wand, J.W.C., (1963) *A History of the Early Church to AD 500,* Methuen, London.

Ward, B. "and Associates" (1996) 2nd edition) *Good Grief: Exploring Feelings, Loss and Death with over 11s and adults,* Jessica Kingsley, London and Bristol.

Ward, C, A., (1989) "Possession and exorcism in magic-religious context" in Ward C.A., ed., (1989) *Altered States of Consciousness and Mental Health,* Sage, London.

Ward, R.H., (1970) "Some aspects of religious life in an immigrant area in Manchester" in Martin and Hill, (1970).

Warrington, K., (2008) *Pentecostal Theology: A Theology of Encounter,* T. & T. Clarke International, London and New York.

Waugh, A., & Grant, A., (2006) *Ross and Wilson's Anatomy and Physiology in health and illness,* 9th Edition, Churchill Livingston Elsevier, Edinburgh, London and New York.

Weber, M., (1947) *The Theory of Social and Economic Organizations*, translated by Henderson, A. & Parsons, T., Oxford University Press, London.

Weber, M., (1968) *Economy and Society*, University of California Press, Los Angeles

Weiss, G. L,. Lonnquist, L. E., (2005) *The Sociology of Health, Healing and Illness*, Pearson Education., Newark, New Jersey.

Wengraf, T., (2001) *Qualitative research: Interviewing, Biographical narrative and Semi-structured methods* Sage, London.

White, K., (2002) *An Introduction to the Sociology of Health and Illness*, Sage, London & New Delhi.

Whitehouse, H., & McCauley, R., (2005) "New Frontiers in the Cognitive Science of Religion" *Journal of Cognition and Culture* Vol. 5 (1-2) pp 1-13.

WHO, (1946) *The Constitution of the World Health Organization*, World Health Organization, Geneva.

WHO, (1992) *The ICD-10 Classification of Mental and Behavioural Disorders*, World Health Organization, Geneva.

Williams, F., (1993) *Social Policy: A Critical Introduction*, Polity Press, Cambridge.

Williams, R., (1958) *Culture and Society*, London, Chatto and Windus.

Winkelman, M., (1998) "Altered States of Consciousness and Religious Behaviour" in Glazier, S., ed., *Anthropology of Religion: A Handbook of Method and Theory*, Greenwood, Westport, Connecticut, pp 393-428.

Winkelman, M., (2000) *Shamanism: The Neural Ecology of Consciousness and Healing*. Bergin and Garvey, Westport, Connecticut.

Winkelman, M., (2001) "Psycho-integrators: Multidisciplinary Perspectives on the Therapeutic Effects of Hallucinogens" *Complementary Health Practice Review* Vol. 6 (3) pp. 219-37.

Winston, B., (2002) *The Spirit of Leadership,* Bill Winston Ministries, Oak Park, Illinois.

Wiseman, R., & Watt C., (2006)" Belief in psychic ability and the misattribution hypothesis: A qualitative review" *British Journal of Psychology* Vol. 97 pp 323-338.

Witvleit, C.van O., Ludwig, T. E., & Vander Laan, K.L., (2001) "Granting forgiveness or harbouring grudges: Implications for emotions, physiology and health" *Journal of Psychological Science* Vol. 12(2) pp 117-123.

Wolcott, H.F., (1990) "On seeking and rejecting validity in qualitative research" in Eisner, H.W., & Peshkin A., eds., *Qualitative Enquiry in Education: The Continuing Absolute,* Teachers College Press, New York.

Wong, Y., and Vinsky, J., (2009) "Speaking from the margins: A critical reflection on the"spiritual-but-not-religious" discourse in social work", *British Journal of Social Work* Vol. 39 (7) pp. 1343-1359.

Wordsworth, H., (2007) "Reclaim the Spirit" *Nursing Standard.* Vol. 22 (10) pp 22-23.

Worthington, E.L., Witvliet, C.van O., Pietrini, P. & Lerner, A.J., (2007) "Forgiveness, health, and well-being: A review of emotional vs decisional forgiveness, dispositional forgivingness and unreduced forgiveness" *Journal of Behavioural Medicine.* Vol. 30 pp 291-302.

Wright, N., & Smith, S., (1997) "A Panorama of Suffering" in Lucas (1997) pp 37-49.

Wright, S., (2007) "The spirit of Good Nursing" *Nursing Standard.* vol. 22 (8) pp 20-21.

Young, F., (1993) *The making of the creeds*, SCM Press, London.

Zizioulas, J., (1985) *Being as Communion: Studies in Personhood and the Church*, St Vladimir's Seminary Contemporary Greek Theologians Series No.4, Crestwood, New York.

Zola, I, K., (1973) "Pathways to the doctor—From Person to Patient" *Social Science and Medicine* Vol.7 (9) pp. 667-89.

Zollinger, T. W., Phillips R., & Kumza J. W., (1984) "Breast Cancer survival rates among Seventh day Adventists and Non-Seventh Day Adventists" *American Journal of Epidemiology* Vol. 119 (4) pp 503-509.

Lightning Source UK Ltd.
Milton Keynes UK
UKOW01f0622081017
310610UK00001B/55/P